Advances in
Epilepsy

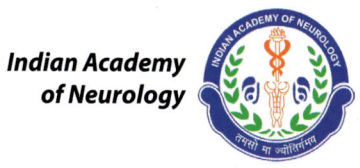

Indian Academy of Neurology

Advances in Epilepsy

Editor-in-Chief

Debashish Chowdhury
DTCD MD(Medicine) DM(Neurology) FIAN FRCP(Edinburgh)
Commonwealth Fellow in Stroke Medicine(Edinburgh)
Director–Professor and Head
Department of Neurology
GB Pant Institute of Postgraduate Medical Education and Research
New Delhi, India

Editors

Sita Jayalakshmi MD DM
Senior Consultant Neurologist
and In-Charge
Comprehensive Epilepsy Care
Programme
Department of Neurology
Krishna Institute of Medical
Sciences
Secunderabad, Telangana, India

Gagandeep Singh DM FAMS FRCP
Professor and Head
Department of Neurology
Dayanand Medical College and
Hospital
Ludhiana, Punjab, India

Sangeeta Ravat MD DM
Professor and Head
Department of Neurology
Dean, Seth GS Medical College
and KEM Hospital
Chief Epileptologist
Comprehensive Epilepsy
Care Centre
KEM Hospital and Global Hospital
Mumbai, Maharashtra, India

Foreword
P Satishchandra

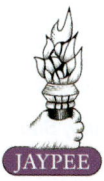

JAYPEE BROTHERS MEDICAL PUBLISHERS
The Health Sciences Publisher
New Delhi | London

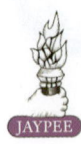

Jaypee Brothers Medical Publishers (P) Ltd

Headquarters
EMCA House
23/23-B, Ansari Road, Daryaganj
New Delhi 110 002, India
Landline: +91-11-23272143, +91-11-23272703
+91-11-23282021, +91-11-23245672
E-mail: jaypee@jaypeebrothers.com

EU GPSR Authorised Representative
Logos Europe, 9 rue Nicolas Poussin
17000, La Rochelle, France
Phone: +33 (0) 6 67 93 73 78
E-mail: Contact@logoseurope.eu

Corporate Office
Jaypee Brothers Medical Publishers (P) Ltd.
4838/24, Ansari Road, Daryaganj
New Delhi 110 002, India
Phone: +91-11-43574357
Fax: +91-11-43574314
E-mail: jaypee@jaypeebrothers.com

Overseas Office
JP Medical Ltd.
83, Victoria Street, London
SW1H 0HW (UK)
Phone: +44-20 3170 8910
Fax: +44(0)20 3008 6180
E-mail: info@jpmedpub.com

Website: www.jaypeebrothers.com
Website: www.jaypeedigital.com

© 2025, Jaypee Brothers Medical Publishers

The views and opinions expressed in this book are solely those of the original contributor(s)/author(s) and do not necessarily represent those of editor(s) or publisher of the book.

All rights reserved. No part of this publication may be reproduced, stored or transmitted in any form or by any means, electronic, mechanical, photocopying, recording or otherwise, without the prior permission in writing of the publishers.

All brand names and product names used in this book are trade names, service marks, trademarks or registered trademarks of their respective owners. The publisher is not associated with any product or vendor mentioned in this book.

Medical knowledge and practice change constantly. This book is designed to provide accurate, authoritative information about the subject matter in question. However, readers are advised to check the most current information available on procedures included and check information from the manufacturer of each product to be administered, to verify the recommended dose, formula, method and duration of administration, adverse effects and contraindications. It is the responsibility of the practitioner to take all appropriate safety precautions. Neither the publisher nor the author(s)/editor(s) assume any liability for any injury and/or damage to persons or property arising from or related to use of material in this book.

This book is sold on the understanding that the publisher is not engaged in providing professional medical services. If such advice or services are required, the services of a competent medical professional should be sought.

Every effort has been made where necessary to contact holders of copyright to obtain permission to reproduce copyright material. If any have been inadvertently overlooked, the publisher will be pleased to make the necessary arrangements at the first opportunity.

Inquiries for bulk sales may be solicited at: jaypee@jaypeebrothers.com

IAN Advances in Epilepsy / Debashish Chowdhury, Sita Jayalakshmi, Gagandeep Singh, Sangeeta Ravat

First Edition: 2025

ISBN: 978-93-6616-814-2

Printed in India at Purewall Ventures Pvt Ltd

Indian Academy of Neurology

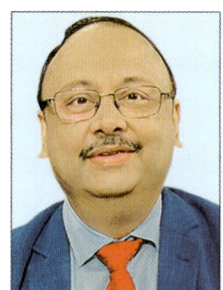

PRESIDENT
Debashish Chowdhury
New Delhi, India

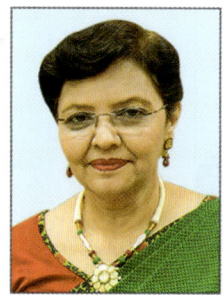

PRESIDENT-ELECT
Sangeeta Ravat
Mumbai, Maharashtra, India

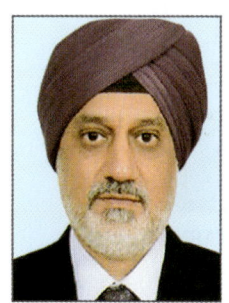

IMMEDIATE PAST PRESIDENT
Gagandeep Singh
Ludhiana, Punjab, India

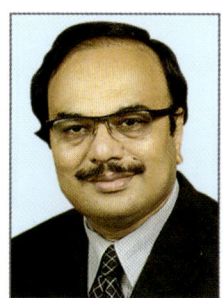

PAST PRESIDENT
Nirmal Surya
Mumbai, Maharashtra, India

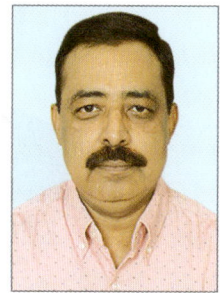

TREASURER
Achal Srivastava
New Delhi, India

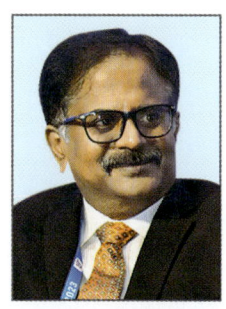

SECRETARY
U Meenakshisundaram
Chennai, Tamil Nadu, India

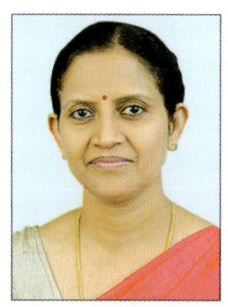

EDITOR, ANNALS OF IAN
PN Sylaja
Thiruvananthapuram, Kerala, India

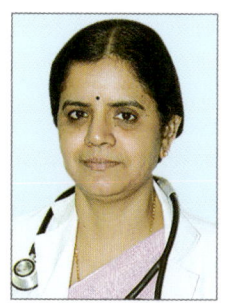

CME CONVENER
Sita Jayalakshmi
Hyderabad, Telangana, India

Executive Members

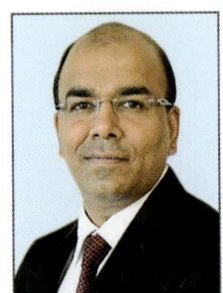

Arvind Sharma
Ahmedabad, Gujarat, India

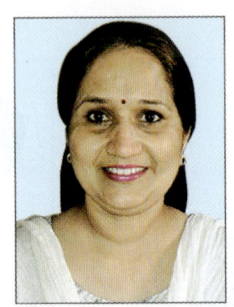

Bhawna Sharma
Jaipur, Rajasthan, India

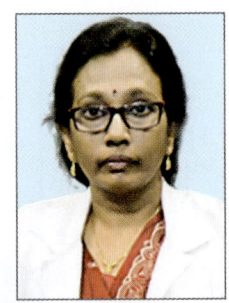

Atchayaram Nalini
Bengaluru, Karnataka, India

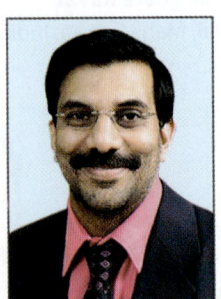

JOINT TREASURER
Pradeep VG
Kozhikode, Kerala, India

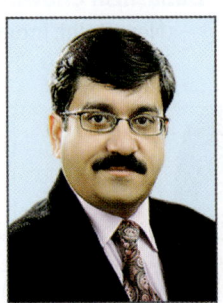

JOINT SECRETARY
Sumit Singh
Gurugram, Haryana, India

Contributors

Abhishek Gohel MBBS
MD(General Medicine) DM
(Neurology) PDF(Epilepsy)
Neurologist and Epileptologist
KD Hospital
Ahmedabad, Gujarat, India

Aditya Sunil Gudhate
DM(Neurology)
Final Year Resident in Neurology
Seth GSMC and KEM Hospital
Mumbai, Maharashtra, India

Anuja Patil MD DM
Consultant Neurologist and
Epileptologist, Krishna Institute
of Medical Sciences
Secunderabad, Telangana, India

Aparna Ramakrishnan MMBS
MD DNB(Psychiatry)
Consultant Psychiatrist
Department of Psychiatry
Kokilaben Dhirubhai Ambani
Hospital and Medical Research
Institute
Mumbai, Maharashtra, India

Ashalatha Radhakrishnan
MD DM
Professor
Chair, Epilepsy Division
R Madhavan Nayar Center for
Comprehensive Epilepsy Care
Sree Chitra Tirunal Institute
for Medical Sciences and
Technology
Thiruvananthapuram, Kerala,
India

Bindu Menon MD(Medicine)
DM(Neurology) DNB(Neurology)
PGDCN(Neurology)(London)
FRCP(Edinburgh) MNAMS FICP FIAN
FWSO FAAN FAMS
Head
Department of Neurology
Apollo Speciality Hospitals
Nellore, Andhra Pradesh, India

Bharat Kumar Sahu MD DM
Senior Resident Neurology
GB Pant Institute of
Postgraduate Medical
Education and Research
New Delhi, India

Bhargavi Sanji MD(Pediatrics)
DM(Pediatric Neurology)
Associate Consultant
Department of Pediatric
Neurology, Manipal Hospitals
Bengaluru, Karnataka, India

Chandu Premkumar
DM(Neurology)
Neurologist and Epileptologist
Rama Chandra Medical College
and Hospital
Chennai, Tamil Nadu, India

Chaturbhuj Rathore MD DM
DNB PDF
Senior Consultant
Department of Neurosciences
Zydus Hospital
Vadodara, Gujarat, India

Dhrumil Shah MBBS MD
DrNB(Neurology)
Consultant Neurologist
CIMS Hospital
Ahmedabad, Gujarat, India

Gagandeep Singh DM FAMS
FRCP
Professor and Head
Department of Neurology
Dayanand Medical College and
Hospital
Ludhiana, Punjab, India

Jayakumari Nandana MD DM
Postdoctoral Fellow
R Madhavan Nayar Center for
Comprehensive Epilepsy Care
Department of Neurology
Sree Chitra Tirunal Institute
for Medical Sciences and
Technology
Thiruvananthapuram, Kerala,
India

Jayanti Mani MBBS MD
DM(Neurology)
Consultant Neurologist
Kokilaben Dhirubhai Ambani
Hospital
Mumbai, Maharashtra, India

Jyotsna AS DNB(Pediatrics)
DM(Pediatric Neurology)
Consultant
Apollo BGS Hospitals
Mysuru, Karnataka, India

KP Vinayan MD DNB DM
Secretary General
Indian Epilepsy Society Chair
Pediatric Neurology Subsection
Indian Academy of Neurology
Associate Editor, Annals of
Indian Academy of Neurology
Secretary
Asian Epilepsy Academy
(ASEPA) Member, Terminology
Commission, ILAE
Professor and Head
Department of Pediatric
Neurology
Amrita Institute of Medical
Sciences
Kochi, Kerala, India

KY Manisha MD DM
Postdoctoral Fellow
R Madhavan Nayar Center for
Comprehensive Epilepsy Care
Department of Neurology
Sree Chitra Tirunal Institute
for Medical Sciences and
Technology
Thiruvananthapuram, Kerala,
India

Manjari Tripathi DM
Professor and Head
Department of Neurology
AIIMS
New Delhi, India

Mehak Arora MBBS MD DM
Senior Resident
Department of Neurology
Dayanand Medical College
Ludhiana, Punjab, India

Parampreet Singh Kharbanda MBBS MD DM
Professor
Department of Neurology
Postgraduate Institute of
Medical Education and
Research
Chandigarh, India

Parthvi Shreyas Ravat MD DrNB(Neurology)
Clinical and Research Fellow
Neuroimmunology Center
for Neuroscience Innovation
Flinders University Adelaide
South Australia

Praveen Kumar Yadav MD DM MRCP(UK) FRCP(Edinburgh) FRCP(London) FEBN(UK)
Senior Consultant Neurologist
Aarogyam Hospital
Durgapur, West Bengal, India

P Sarat Chandra MCH
Professor
Department of Neurosurgery
AIIMS
New Delhi, India

Rutul Shah MBBS DNB DM(Neurology) MNAMS PDF(Epilepsy)
Consultant Neurologist and
Epileptologist
KD Hospital
Ahmedabad, Gujarat, India

Sangeeta Ravat MD DM
Professor and Head
Department of Neurology
Dean, Seth GS Medical College
and KEM Hospital
Chief Epileptologist
Comprehensive Epilepsy
Care Centre, KEM Hospital and
Global Hospital
Mumbai, Maharashtra, India

Siby Gopinath MD(General Medicine) DNB(Neurology) MNAMS
Professor of Neurology
Amrita Institute of Medical
Sciences
Kochi, Kerala, India

Sita Jayalakshmi MD DM
Senior Consultant Neurologist
and In-Charge
Comprehensive Epilepsy Care
Programme
Department of Neurology
Krishna Institute of Medical
Sciences
Secunderabad, Telangana, India

Swapan Gupta MD DM
Associate Professor
Department of Neurology
GB Pant Institute of
Postgraduate Medical
Education and Research
New Delhi, India

S Sidharth MD
Senior Resident
Department of Neurology
AIIMS
New Delhi, India

Foreword

Epilepsy is the second most common neurological disorder with almost 14 million people living with epilepsy in India, not sparing any specific age-group. Rapid advances are happening in the understanding and management of epilepsy in the last two decades. It is essential to have a book on *"Advances in Epilepsy"*. I am very happy to note that the Indian Academy of Neurology (IAN) has taken the responsibility to disseminate the recent information on the management of epilepsy by publishing a book on this topic in 2024.

This book is a multiauthored book published by Jaypee Brothers Medical Publishers which includes 12 chapters. The editor has chosen the most important topics, starting from the management of the first unprovoked seizure, which has been extensively studied in these two decades. It has been emphasized that the risk of recurrence is higher in the first 2 years, but a single unprovoked seizure does not affect the long-term outcome of epilepsy. Medical management of epilepsy has two important chapters: One discussing the art and science of choosing antiseizure medications, emphasizing the role of monotherapy, and the other laying emphasis on the role of rational polytherapy in the management of drug-resistant epilepsy (DRE). There are two chapters discussing the role of antiseizure medications (ASMs) in special population: Women and elderly. With the changing demographic in this country, one needs to be aware about how to manage epilepsy in these two special population categories. This remains a challenge. The chapter on genetics of epilepsy targets "Precision Medicine" especially in children with epilepsy syndromes.

This book has two chapters on nonmedical management of epilepsy, including the role of surgery in remedial epilepsy and palliation. The author clearly characterized Level I Center and Level II Center. I found this as extremely important to recognize before contemplating surgery in any center in this country, which should be based on the resources available thus aiming at improving the quality of life of these unfortunate people with epilepsy. The chapter on neurostimulation highlights the role of vagus nerve stimulation (VNS), responsive neurostimulation (RNS), and deep brain stimulation (DBS). But unfortunately, VNS is getting out of practice globally and RNS has still not entered this country. However, neurostimulation in epilepsy is very important, especially for those with DRE where surgery is not a possible solution.

Other chapters include criteria for withdrawing ASMs, which discuss about prediction models and online models but clearly state that ASM can be successfully withdrawn in only 30–40% patients. This chapter has brought out the latest information that even among IGE, in selected cases, drug can be withdrawn. This needs to be cautiously observed and requires further follow-up. This book is written in a very simple language. It is well researched and has the latest references, even up to 2022/2023, and hence will be extremely useful for postgraduate students and also practicing neurologists and neurosurgeons interested in the field of epilepsy.

I wish the editor would have included a chapter on the management of "Status Epilepsy", and not only Refractory Status Epilepticus, and another on the classification of epilepsy in 2024 as the International League Against Epilepsy (ILAE) is seriously considering bringing out a new classification of epilepsy and epilepsy syndrome in the coming year. Overall, I congratulate the IAN for bringing out this book on "Advances in Epilepsy", which is very timely and should be in every library. I am sure IAN will bring out a soft version of this book which can be used on the bedside by postgraduates and practicing neurologists.

P Satishchandra
MBBS DM(Neurology) DSc(Hon) FAMS FRCP(London) FIAN FKST
President, Indian Epilepsy Association
Senior Consultant, Apollo Speciality Hospitals
Former Director and Vice Chancellor, NIMHANS
Bengaluru, Karnataka, India

Message from Editor-in-Chief

Dear Readers,

The Indian Academy of Neurology (IAN) has been at the forefront of neurology education and has a rich history of publications which rank high in terms of academic and scientific content. As President, it has been my pleasure to team up with my Executive Committee members, who are experts in various neurological subspecialties and high-quality and prolific authors with an impressive track record of publications, as editors and bring out a series of books which continue to hold high the tradition of IAN in terms of high-impact scientific content.

As Chief Editor of IAN *"Advances in Epilepsy"*, it is my pleasure to bring to you a book which sets the bar high for content—accurate, updated, and relevant—and at the same time presents it in a reader-friendly manner, which makes the book an ideal companion for everyone interested in the subject. I thank my colleagues and editors of this book, *Dr Sita Jayalakshmi, Dr Gagandeep Singh and Dr Sangeeta Ravat*, for the shared vision of high-quality, focused content as well as excellent support rendered during the making of this book.

This has been our collective effort, and we sincerely hope that each of you will like reading this book as much as we loved bringing this out.

Debashish Chowdhury

Preface

Epilepsy is a complex disorder that affects people of all ages. Around 50 million people worldwide have epilepsy and nearly 80% of people with epilepsy live in low- and middle-income countries. The diagnosis and management of epilepsy need great care and the selection of antiseizure medication needs to be individualized with the availability of many newer antiseizure drugs. Nearly one third of people with epilepsy do not respond to antiseizure medications; surgery will help to reduce or eliminate seizures in properly selected people with drug-resistant epilepsy.

This book *"IAN Advances in Epilepsy"* collates state-of-the-art diagnostic and therapeutic developments in the management of epilepsy. We are confident that this compilation will be of immense value to neurologists and physicians dealing with persons with epilepsy.

Sita Jayalakshmi
Gagandeep Singh
Sangeeta Ravat

Acknowledgments

As the editors of the book *"IAN Advances in Epilepsy"*, we feel immensely happy that we had the opportunity to contribute for the academic activities of the Indian Academy of Neurology (IAN). This was a gratifying experience.

First of all, we are extremely grateful to all the eminent authors for submitting the chapters in a restricted time and meticulously preparing the manuscripts. We sincerely thank Dr Debashish Chowdhury, the President, Dr U Meenakshisundaram, the Secretary, and all the executive committee members of IAN for their constant support during the preparation of this book.

We thank the publication team at M/s Jaypee Brothers Medical Publishers (P) Ltd—Ms Chetna Malhotra (Senior Director—Professional Publishing, Marketing and Business Development) and Mr Prashant Mahajan (Development Editor)—for their professional approach and support in bringing out this compilation.

Sita Jayalakshmi
Gagandeep Singh
Sangeeta Ravat

Contents

CHAPTER 1:	**Management of First Unprovoked Seizure** *Dhrumil Shah, Anuja Patil, Sita Jayalakshmi*	1
CHAPTER 2:	**Epilepsy in Older People** *Mehak Arora, Gagandeep Singh*	9
CHAPTER 3:	**Management of Women with Epilepsy** *Parthvi Shreyas Ravat, Aditya Sunil Gudhate, Sangeeta Ravat*	17
CHAPTER 4:	**The Art and Science of Choosing and Combining Antiseizure Medications** *Parampreet Singh Kharbanda*	30
CHAPTER 5:	**Medical Management of Drug-resistant Epilepsy** *Bharat Kumar Sahu, Swapan Gupta*	40
CHAPTER 6:	**Withdrawing Antiseizure Medicines in Seizure Free Patients: Challenges and Solutions** *Chaturbhuj Rathore*	48
CHAPTER 7:	**Management of Surgically Remediable Epilepsy** *S Sidharth, P Sarat Chandra, Manjari Tripathi*	62
CHAPTER 8:	**Neurostimulation in Epilepsy** *Siby Gopinath, Rutul Shah, Abhishek Gohel*	78
CHAPTER 9:	**Management of Refractory Status Epilepticus** *Jayakumari Nandana, KY Manisha, Ashalatha Radhakrishnan*	93
CHAPTER 10:	**Management of Functional Seizures** *Jayanti Mani, Aparna Ramakrishnan*	109

CHAPTER 11:	**Management of Genetic Epilepsies**	122
	Jyotsna AS, Bhargavi Sanji, KP Vinayan	
CHAPTER 12:	**Management of Comorbidities of Epilepsy**	130
	Bindu Menon, Chandu Premkumar, Praveen Kumar Yadav	

Index   141

Management of First Unprovoked Seizure

Dhrumil Shah, Anuja Patil, Sita Jayalakshmi

ABSTRACT

First seizure carries a profound impact on personal, social, and professional aspects of a person. It is important to evaluate it to confirm and assess the risk of recurrence of seizures in the future. Thorough history, analysis of semiology, clinical examination, and basic investigations including electrocardiogram, blood glucose, and electrolytes help to rule out seizure mimics like syncope, hypoglycemia, tetany, or other nonepileptic events. It may also bring into consideration, previous unnoticed myoclonic jerks, nocturnal tongue bites, absences, or hypomotor seizures, thus helping to confirm etiology in otherwise first clinical seizure. An electroencephalogram (EEG) performed within 48 hours of presentation with a seizure increases the yield to detect abnormalities up to almost 70%. In cases with potentially focal clinical onset or other correlating features like postictal deficits and focal EEG abnormalities, imaging features may help in further confirming the etiology and risk of recurrence. Focal onset seizures, multiple seizures at onset or status epilepticus as first episode, clinical neuro-deficits, previous insults including perinatal complications, developmental delay, and abnormal EEG or imaging features carry a higher chance of recurrence, therefore impacting the decision to treat. The risk of recurrence is highest in the first 2 years after the first episode. Although immediate treatment after a first seizure only prevents early risk of recurrence, it does not affect long-term seizure outcome. Choice of antiseizure medication (ASM) depends on age, gender, seizure type, and associated comorbidities. Often creating a lot of concern and a state of panic after a first unprovoked seizure, the family should be counseled about the risk of recurrence, identifying future episodes, need for treatment and compliance, efficacy of treatment, precautions while driving, and social impact.

Keywords: First seizure, Unprovoked seizure, Recurrence, Epilepsy, Treatment.

INTRODUCTION

Overall, at least 10% of the population will get a seizure at some point in their lives.[1] However, only 2–3% of these go on to develop epilepsy later.[2] The first seizure episode carries a significant impact on personal, social, and professional aspects of life. It is vital to evaluate thoroughly but not overzealously, to ascertain the diagnosis of a seizure, estimate the risk of recurrence, need for appropriate treatment, and future implications.

In 2014, International League Against Epilepsy (ILAE) proposed an operational clinical definition for epilepsy as at least two unprovoked seizures occurring >24 hours apart or one unprovoked seizure with an equivalent risk (at least 60%) of recurrence over the next 10 years or diagnosis of epilepsy syndrome.[3] Diagnosis of first seizure and its likelihood of recurrence is important in the decision to start as well as the duration of treatment. Apart from the clinical aspects, it also impacts social domains, including education, driving, career, and marital and family planning. Therefore, when a person comes with first seizure to the clinic, the following questions need to be addressed:

- Is it really a seizure?
- If yes, then is it an acute symptomatic seizure (ASS) or unprovoked seizure (US)?
- If US, then what are the chances of recurrence?
- Do we need to start treatment after first seizure?
- Will starting the treatment early influence the long-term prognosis?
- What should one do if "this" happens again?

■ FIRST TRANSIENT NEUROLOGIC EVENT: IS IT A SEIZURE?

Description of the event or semiology is crucial in diagnosing the seizure. Clinician hardly ever witnesses a seizure and the patient is often not aware during the event. This makes diagnosis difficult by relying on the parts described by the witnesses. Although the dawn of smartphone era has seemingly proved helpful in cases where the event is likely captured in homemade videos; the panic of an unforeseen occurrence of the seizure for the first time, makes it difficult for the family members to video-record the event. The likely focal onset that may precede some generalized seizures might sometimes be missed. Likewise, sometimes myoclonus of limbs in generalized seizures may be interpreted as focal.

Asking the patient, if the aura was present, can give a clue to the event. The prodromal symptoms like lightheadedness, sweating, or visual disturbance prior to losing consciousness favor syncope. Asking the witness about history like stiffness of the body, deviation of the eyes, and drooling may help. Postictal confusion if noticed can help to differentiate seizure from syncope. On examination, tongue bite (especially lateral), posterior dislocation of shoulder, or burns during the event are reliable signs of seizures.[3,4] Urine incontinence or some injuries during the event are more suggestive of seizures but may be noted at times in psychogenic nonepileptic seizures (PNES).[4,5]

With careful history and examination, we need to rule out seizure mimics carefully. One study reported that around 17% of the patients arriving at clinic after the first seizure actually had seizure mimic episodes of other etiology. Most common mimics among them were reflex syncope and PNES.[6] Such common mimicking events are syncope, psychiatric disturbances (dissociative disorder, PNES, or panic attack), transient ischemic attack, transient global amnesia, migraine with brainstem aura, sleep disorders, intoxication of substances, or drugs, etc. Syncope may present with prominent motor movements as convulsive syncope.

Detailed symptomology may help in recognizing unnoticed ictal episodes in the past as well. Previous myoclonic jerks on awakening, tongue bites in sleep, brief absences, or unaware automatisms interpreted as behavioral stereotypies may help in diagnosing likely idiopathic generalized epilepsy or focal onset hypomotor epilepsy in patients seeking medical aid after "first" noticeable seizure.

■ EVALUATING THE TYPE OF SEIZURE: ACUTE SYMPTOMATIC SEIZURE OR UNPROVOKED SEIZURE?

Unprovoked seizures are the ones that occur without any causative acute clinical condition, or they occur outside the interval of defined ASS. While ASS occur due to systemic disorders like metabolic derangements, drug/toxin exposure, or alcohol or substance intoxication or withdrawal, they also occur in the setting of acute brain insult like ischemic stroke, hemorrhage, traumatic brain injury (TBI), central nervous system (CNS) infection, hypoxic brain injury, etc. Seizure occurring within 1 week of CNS insult or during the active phase of infection are called ASS and those occurring later or after the active phase of initial insult are called remote symptomatic seizures.[7]

Differentiation among them is important as there is a difference in recurrence, mortality, and management between ASS and US. Hesdorffer et al. described that higher mortality is noted among the patients with ASS compared to US with a relative risk of 8.9 [95% confidence interval (CI) 3.5–22.5] within 30 days while those who survive 30 days have lower 10-year mortality compared to US.[8] After acute brain insult and ASS, the chances are higher for development of remote symptomatic seizure or epilepsy later.[9]

Clinical evaluation with an electrocardiogram (ECG) helps to detect cardiac arrhythmias or any structural causes that may present with convulsive syncope with very brief prodrome or may even cause ASS. Sometimes laboratory markers like lactate, creatine kinase, and prolactin levels can be done in postictal state in unwitnessed episodes as they are elevated in bilateral tonic–clonic seizures (BTCS). But none of these markers reliably confirm or rule out the diagnosis of seizure.[10] Laboratory evaluation in suspected first ASS include electrolytes, glucose, calcium, magnesium, renal and liver function tests, and complete blood count.[11] Screening for drug abuse is done when previous intake is suggestive. Lumbar puncture should be considered only in suspected cases of CNS infection.

Studies recommend emergent neuroimaging [computed tomography (CT) or magnetic resonance imaging (MRI)] in all patients with first seizure.[12,13] American Academy of Neurology (AAN) reviewed the studies of imaging in 1st seizure and found out that nonenhanced CT brain changed management in 9–17% cases in adults and 3–8% cases in children.[13] Due to wide availability and lower cost, CT is used more often but MRI is more sensitive and superior in giving information for evaluation, especially in conditions like dysplastic cortex. So, MRI, if available, is preferred over CT if there are no contraindications.

Management of ASS generally includes treating the underlying disease, but if patient is having recurrent seizures or status epilepticus, antiseizure medication (ASM) use is advised.[14,15]

■ EVALUATION FOR UNPROVOKED SEIZURE

When after a thorough history, general, neurological examination, and necessary evaluation do not reveal any likely provoking factors for a first seizure, it is considered to be unprovoked. Next evaluation will focus on the type of seizure. If witnessed BTCS, then any focal findings noticed before secondary generalization or myoclonic jerks experienced before seizure should be asked. Apart from the present seizure, any other seizure type experienced by patient such as myoclonic jerks or absences should be specifically enquired. If any focal motor or nonmotor seizures were noticed previously by family, it can help in further localizing the seizure. While evaluating patients with first seizure, 39–52% had been shown to have a history of previous unrecognized seizures.[6,16]

History of previous birth insult or delayed development may help in early-onset epilepsies. History of previous febrile seizures, CNS insult, or childhood trauma can be helpful. Family history is also important, especially in genetic epilepsies like juvenile myoclonic epilepsy. Focal neuro-deficits may indicate structural lesion.

American Academy of Neurology recommends electroencephalogram (EEG) and neuroimaging in all cases of adults with first US (class B).[17] EEG is not performed in emergency unless indicated. Yield of EEG showing significant abnormality when performed on out-patient basis is around 29% according to various studies.[17] The best timing of the EEG is still not clear after 1st seizure but if performed within 48 hours of seizure then yield can increase up to 70.7% as per 1 study.[18] But, immediately after seizure, EEG may show postictal slowing, which is of uncertain significance.

An EEG recording in drowsiness and sleep increases the yield of epileptiform abnormalities. Therefore, a sleep-deprived EEG has better yield than a routine EEG. Epileptiform discharges are associated with a higher risk of recurrence of seizure as compared to normal.[17] Finding epileptiform abnormality also helps in classifying the seizure into focal or generalized, though normal EEG does not rule out diagnosis of epilepsy.

Abnormal neuroimaging carries a higher likelihood of recurrence. According to an analysis by ILAE subcommittee on pediatric neuroimaging guidelines, nearly 50% of neuroimaging studies are found to be abnormal in children presenting with new-onset epilepsy or seizures.[19] Among adults presenting with new-onset seizures, potentially epileptogenic lesions were found in nearly 28% of cases.[20] Although lesions like mesial temporal sclerosis, focal cortical dysplasia, tumors, and vascular malformations are known to be associated with epilepsy, sometimes imaging may be misleading with incidental focal calcifications, developmental vascular anomalies, or other likely benign lesions. Therefore, in cases with potentially focal clinical onset or other correlating features like postictal deficits, focal EEG abnormalities and imaging features may help in further confirming the etiology and risk of recurrence.

■ RISK OF RECURRENCE AFTER FIRST UNPROVOKED SEIZURE

After initial evaluation, the next step will be assessing the risk of recurrence, and thereby deciding the need for future treatment and follow-up. As discussed, the risk of recurrence is lower in ASS and the risk of short-term mortality is higher, while in cases of remote symptomatic seizure that occur after 1 week of acute brain insult, the risk of recurrence is higher. One study showed that the risk of recurrence in the future is around 33% if seizure happens within 1 week of acute ischemic stroke while the recurrence risk is 71.5% if any seizure occurs after 1 week of stroke.[8] Same study shows the risk of seizure recurrence of 13.4% in acute phase of TBI while late seizure has 46% recurrence risk.[8] Similarly, risk of recurrence is higher with previous history of CNS infection or neonatal brain injury. These patients have higher chances of developing subsequent epilepsy.

One prospective study of 208 patients with 1st US evaluated that the risk of recurrence is 14%, 29%, and 34% at 1, 3, and 5 years respectively.[21] Among these, patients with remote symptomatic seizures have almost 2.5 times risk of recurrence whereas in those with idiopathic seizures, the risk factors were sibling with epilepsy, generalized spike-wave discharges in EEG, and history of ASS.[21] The MESS trial (Multicenter trial for Early epilepsy and Single Seizure) made a prognostic model to identify patients with low, moderate, and high risk of seizure recurrence. They identified that patients with abnormal EEG, any neurological disorder (focal deficits, developmental delay, learning disabilities, etc.), or multiple (two or three) seizures are at moderate risk. Patients with the presence of two of these features or more than three seizures are at higher risk, and those with a history of one seizure without any of these features are at lower risk of recurrence.[22] Occurrence of status epilepticus or multiple seizures as first unprovoked event often merits treatment with ASMs. Although the literature varies since some studies exclude status epilepticus in assessing the risk of recurrence.[23]

Though most studies were conducted on the adult population, one prospective study in children showed that the risk of recurrence after the first unprovoked afebrile seizure was 29%, 37%, 42%, and 44% at 1, 2, 5, and 8 years, respectively. Risk factors for recurrence in children are remote symptomatic etiology, abnormal EEG, seizure in sleep, history of febrile seizure, and postictal Todd's paresis.[24] Focal seizures have a higher risk of recurrence compared to generalized seizures since they are most often associated with structural etiology, abnormal focal EEG, or imaging features.

Timing of recurrence is also of importance for continuing treatment. Both adult and pediatric studies showed that the risk of recurrence is highest in first 2 years. In the pediatric study, the median time for recurrence was 5.7 months and 88% of patients had recurrence within 2 years.[24] While adult studies also showed highest recurrence within 2 years of 1st US.[21,25]

■ STARTING ANTISEIZURE MEDICATIONS AFTER FIRST UNPROVOKED SEIZURE

The decision to treat with ASMs depends upon the likelihood of recurrence of seizures after first US, which is estimated by the clinical, neuroimaging, and EEG analysis. After the first US, usually, no immediate treatment is required, if EEG and neuroimaging are normal. In cases of provoked seizures (electrolyte imbalance and toxin exposure), only treatment of the underlying condition is advised rather than prophylactic ASM. If the child is suspected to have self-limiting epilepsy [e.g., self-limited epilepsy with centrotemporal spikes (SeLECTS)] then only monitoring of seizures is warranted.

In case of a BTCS or loss of consciousness with an actual or potential risk of injury, aggressive treatment is required compared to focal nondisabling seizures. The treatment options are also influenced by other factors like women in reproductive age, comorbidities and consequential polypharmacy, old age (more risk of side effects), occupation, and driving privileges (adults).

Another factor in treatment comprises the optimal duration. According to FIRST study, the risk of occurrence of a second seizure was 26% in the immediately-treated group and 45% in delayed-treated group. But seizure remission rate was similar in the arms at first and second year of follow-up.[23] The MESS trial also showed starting the treatment after first BTCS will delay the next seizure but long-term seizure freedom is not affected.[25] **Flowchart 1** summarizes the approach to first seizure.

The AAN 2015 guideline for unprovoked first seizure in adults recommends few points to be considered in counseling of the patient/relative before considering ASM. Risk of recurrence of seizures is highest in first 2 years (21–45%). Immediate start of ASM when compared to delayed start will likely reduce the occurrence of second seizure but may not improve quality of life. Immediate treatment is unlikely to improve long-term prognosis in achieving seizure freedom compared to delay in treatment. The risk of side effects of ASM is around 7–31%, but these are mostly mild and reversible.[26]

Choosing the first ASM after first US depends on many factors like comorbidities, age of the patient, childbearing potential, etc.

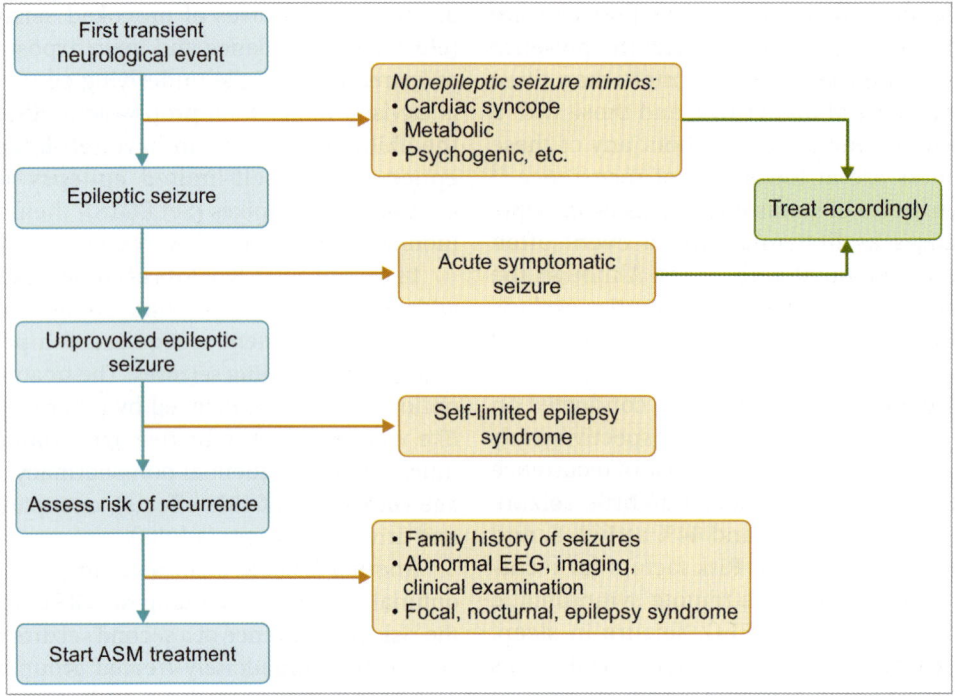

FLOWCHART 1: Approach to first seizure.
(ASM: antiseizure medication; EEG: electroencephalogram)

Detailed description of ASM is out the scope of this chapter. In some comorbid conditions like migraine (topiramate) or depression (lamotrigine), ASM with dual benefits can be useful. Enzyme-inducing ASMs (phenytoin, carbamazepine, lamotrigine, etc.) should be used with caution in patients who are on vitamin K antagonists or women on oral contraceptives. Some medications have better side effect profile compared to others, especially the second-generation ASMs are preferred over first due to better tolerability. When lamotrigine, gabapentin, and carbamazepine were used as first-line ASM in elderly, lamotrigine or gabapentin had lower side effects and higher retention compared to carbamazepine.[27] Choice of ASM also varies according to the type of seizures (focal vs. generalized). Patients with genetic generalized epilepsy will benefit from broad-spectrum ASMs. If the exact type of seizure is not known, then also a broad-spectrum ASM is a better choice. ASMs like lamotrigine and perampanel need to be titrated slowly over weeks compared to levetiracetam and lacosamide, which attains their therapeutic level quickly.

■ COUNSELING AFTER FIRST SEIZURE

Management of seizure does not end with medical treatment. First seizure creates a lot of apprehension regarding the event, possible etiology, risk of developing a seizure again, and need for treatment. Decision to treat should be made by including patient/relative in decision-making, and explaining benefits and adverse events of ASMs. Family should be counseled on how to recognize seizures and what to do if an aura occurs. They should be educated regarding the likelihood of seizures precipitated by sleep deprivation, noncompliance with ASM, or during illness and intoxication. Seizure first aid must be explained, especially in cases of BTCS to family or coworkers. Person should be explained about driving restrictions after the first seizure. Counseling regarding sudden unexpected death in epilepsy (SUDEP) should be done. Stigma and psychiatric comorbidity related to epilepsy need to be addressed.[11,28]

CONCLUSION

People with suspected first seizures should be evaluated by careful detailed history and investigation to confirm the "first" event and that the event was "epileptic" in nature. ASS should be identified and treated accordingly. EEG and neuroimaging should be performed in cases as per the indication. Treatment is usually recommended after two USs or after the first US and higher (>60%) risk of recurrence. ASM choice depends on age, gender, seizure type, and associated comorbidities. Counseling of the family should be done in all cases of the first seizure.

REFERENCES

1. Berg AT, Shinnar S. The risk of seizure recurrence following a first unprovoked seizure: A quantitative review. Neurology. 1991;41(7):965-72.
2. Hauser WA, Beghi E. First seizure definitions and worldwide incidence and mortality. Epilepsia. 2008;49(Supp1):8-12.
3. Fisher RS, Acevedo C, Arzimanoglou A, Bogacz A, Cross JH, Elger CE, et al. ILAE official report: A practical clinical definition of epilepsy. Epilepsia. 2014;55(4):475-82.
4. Peguero E, Abou-Khalil B, Fakhoury T, Mathews G. Self-injury and incontinence in psychogenic seizures. Epilepsia. 1995;36(6):586-91.
5. Dworetzky BA, Weisholtz DS, Perez DL, Baslet G. A clinically oriented perspective on psychogenic nonepileptic seizure–related emergencies. Clin EEG Neurosci. 2015;46(1):26-33.
6. Jackson A, Teo L, Seneviratne U. Challenges in the first seizure clinic for adult patients with epilepsy. Epileptic Disord. 2016;18(3):305-14.
7. Beghi E, Carpio A, Forsgren L, Hesdorffer DC, Malmgren K, Sander JW, et al. Recommendation for a definition of acute symptomatic seizure. Epilepsia. 2010;51(4):671-5.
8. Hesdorffer DC, Benn EK, Cascino GD, Hauser WA. Is a first acute symptomatic seizure epilepsy? Mortality and risk for recurrent seizure. Epilepsia. 2009;50(5):1102-8.
9. Herman ST. Epilepsy after brain insult: Targeting epileptogenesis. Neurology. 2002;59(9):S21-6.
10. Nass RD, Sassen R, Elger CE, Surges R. The role of postictal laboratory blood analyses in the diagnosis and prognosis of seizures. Seizure. 2017;47:51-65.
11. Epilepsies: Diagnosis and management (NICE). London: National Institute for Health and Care Excellence (NICE); 2021.
12. Kotisaari K, Virtanen P, Forss N, Strbian D, Scheperjans J. Emergency computed tomography in patients with first seizure. Seizure. 2017;48: 89-93.
13. Harden CL, Huff JS, Schwartz TH, Dubinsky RM, Zimmerman RD, Weinstein S, et al. Reassessment: Neuroimaging in the emergency patient presenting with seizure (an evidence-based review): Report of the therapeutics and technology assessment subcommittee of the American Academy of Neurology. Neurology. 2007;69(18):1772-80.
14. Hesdorffer DC, Logroscino G, Cascino G, Annegers JF, Hauser WA. Risk of unprovoked seizure after acute symptomatic seizure: Effect of status epilepticus. Ann Neurol. 1998;44(6):908-12.
15. Leung H, Man CB, Hui AC, Kwan P, Wong KS. Prognosticating acute symptomatic seizures using two different seizure outcomes. Epilepsia. 2010;51(8):1570-9.
16. Jallon P, Loiseau P, Loiseau J. Newly diagnosed unprovoked epileptic seizures: Presentation at diagnosis in CAROLE study. Coordination

Active du Réseau Observatoire Longitudinal de l' Epilepsie. Epilepsia. 2001;42(4):464-75.
17. Krumholz A, Wiebe S, Gronseth G, Shinnar S, Levisohn P, Ting T, et al. Practice parameter: Evaluating an apparent unprovoked first seizure in adults (an evidence-based review): Report of the Quality Standards Subcommittee of the American Academy of Neurology and the American Epilepsy Society. Neurology. 2007;69(21):1996-2007.
18. Schreiner A, Pohlmann-Eden B. Value of the early electroencephalogram after a first unprovoked seizure. Clin Electroencephalogr. 2003;34(3):140-4.
19. Gaillard WD, Chiron C, Cross JH, Harvey AS, Kuzniecky R, Hertz-Pannier, L, et al. Guidelines for imaging infants and children with recent-onset epilepsy. Epilepsia. 2009;50(9):2147-53.
20. Hakami T, McIntosh A, Todaro M, Lui E, Yerra R, Tan KM, et al. MRI-identified pathology in adults with new-onset seizures. Neurology. 2013;81(10): 920-7.
21. Hauser WA, Rich SS, Annegers JF, Anderson VE. Seizure recurrence after a 1st unprovoked seizure: An extended follow-up. Neurology. 1990; 40(8):1163-70.
22. Kim LG, Johnson TL, Marson AG, Chadwick DW; MRC MESS Study group. Prediction of risk of seizure recurrence after a single seizure and early epilepsy: Further results from the MESS trial. Lancet Neurol. 2006;5(4):317-22.
23. Musicco M, Beghi E, Solari A, Viani F. Treatment of first tonic–clonic seizure does not improve the prognosis of epilepsy. First Seizure Trial Group (FIRST Group). Neurology. 1997;49(4):991-8
24. Shinnar S, Berg AT, Moshe SL, O'Dell C, Alemany M, Newstein D. The risk of seizure recurrence after a first unprovoked afebrile seizure in childhood: An extended follow-up. Pediatrics. 1996;98 (2 Pt 1):216-25.
25. Marson A, Jacoby A, Johnson A, Kim L, Gamble C, Chadwick D. Immediate versus deferred antiepileptic drug treatment for early epilepsy and single seizures: A randomised controlled trial. Lancet. 2005;365(9476):2007-13.
26. Krumholz A, Wiebe S, Gronseth GS, Gloss DS, Sanchez AM, Kabir AA, et al. Evidence-based guideline: Management of an unprovoked first seizure in adults: Report of the Guideline Development Subcommittee of the American Academy of Neurology and the American Epilepsy Society. Neurology. 2015;84(16):1705-13.
27. Rowan AJ, Ramsay RE, Collins JF, Pryor F, Boardman KD, Uthman BM, et al. New onset geriatric epilepsy: A randomized study of gabapentin, lamotrigine, and carbamazepine. Neurology. 2005;64(11):1868-73.
28. Legg KT, Newton M. Counselling adults who experience a first seizure. Seizure. 2017;49:64-8.

CHAPTER 2

Epilepsy in Older People

Mehak Arora, Gagandeep Singh

ABSTRACT

The occurrence of seizures and epilepsy in older people is under recognized and often ignored. People older than 60 years are at increased risk of both new-onset acute symptomatic as well as unprovoked seizures. The etiology of seizures in the elderly includes cerebrovascular diseases, neurodegenerative conditions—in particular dementia of Alzhiemer's disease, traumatic brain injury, metabolic abnormalities, and drugs. Seizures may merely present with altered mental status, confusional episodes, or wandering episodes, or just memory disturbance unlike the typical sensorimotor semiologies in the younger individuals. In older people, auras are much less frequent, if at all present as generally nonspecific (e.g., dizziness), not allowing it to be of localizing value. Automatisms are likewise less frequent in older adults. On the contrary, postictal confusion can be considerably prolonged such that the older people with epilepsy can stay drowsy or confused up to days following a seizure episode. The differential diagnosis for epilepsy is broad in the elderly and includes syncope, metabolic disturbances, transient ischemic attacks, cardiac events or arrhythmias, sleep disorders including rapid eye movement (REM)-sleep behavior disorder, and psychogenic nonepileptic seizures. Levetiracetam, lacosamide, and brivaracetam are recommended for the management of epilepsy in the elderly.

Keywords: Epilepsy, Elderly, Cerebrovascular accidents, Dementia, Antiseizure medications.

■ INTRODUCTION

Seizures and epilepsy can occur at any age but it is often thought that these typically occur in younger people. The occurrence of seizures and epilepsy in older people is unrecognized and often ignored. In this chapter, we hope to convince readers that, not only are seizures and epilepsy common in older people but also merit special attention and consideration over and above epilepsy in other age groups. Seizures and epilepsy in older people merit special and specific considerations among the epileptologists and neurologists in terms of etiology, choice of treatment, pharmacokinetics, including drug–drug interactions, pharmacodynamic, and adverse effects profile. Of note, recent epidemiological studies from western, high income countries suggest a significant rise in the incidence and prevalence of epilepsy in the elderly population as well as a decline in the incidence of epilepsy in extremely young people. Moreover, people aged older than 65 years represent the fastest growing age group globally. The account here, in this chapter, with its factual and conceptual detail is a call to pay more attention to the study of seizures and epilepsy in older people.

■ EPIDEMIOLOGY

There is irrefutable evidence that people older than 60 years are at increased risk of both new-onset acute symptomatic as well as unprovoked seizures.[1] A bimodal peak of the age-specific incidence of epilepsy was established in early population-based epidemiological studies from Rochester, USA and confirmed later in other geographic locations.[2] The age-specific incidence of epilepsy follows a "U" shaped curve with peaks at the two extremes of life, i.e., very young infants and children and the older people. Of note, more recent population-based epidemiological studies from western high-income countries have suggested that the early life peak is diminishing, on account of better pre- and perinatal care, and a reduction in the incidence of central nervous system infections, whilst the late-life peak is increasing on account of greater longevity of populations. As well as, the increasing access to medical care, better comorbidity awareness and management among older people has also contributed to the increasing late-life peak. There is a parallel increase in aging-related epileptogenic substrates, such as stroke and Alzheimer's disease (AD). This trend in demographics is only expected to continue to increase in this direction.[3] Whether these demographic attributes apply to the Indian context as well is unclear, as there are very limited studies of the age-specific incidence of epilepsy from India. High-quality, population-based studies are difficult to conduct in the given environment but are really desirable. At the same time, there are not many clinic-based studies of older people with epilepsy from within the country. This may give, perhaps the mistaken impression that epilepsy is not common in older people. It is however, likely, that older people and seizures and epilepsy do not present to medical attention as the symptoms and signs are often ignored or unrecognized. Older people also face difficulties in presenting to hospital on account of poor ambulation and independence.

Besides, epilepsy, older people also experience acute symptomatic seizures more commonly in comparison to relatively younger people. This is perhaps on account of the increased incidence of proximate brain insults in this age group, e.g., stroke, metabolic disorders, etc. Overall, the cumulative prevalence of epilepsy increases with advancing age but the age-specific prevalence of epilepsy in older people might not be commensurately high. This is because many epilepsies acquired in younger ages remit and some people with epilepsy that onsets in the younger age might die prematurely. For new-onset epilepsies in the older people, the years lived with disability as well as years of life lost might be comparatively smaller in comparison to early-onset epilepsies. There is, however, one distinct subgroup of epilepsies in older people, i.e., those who have epilepsy with onset in young age and grow in to old age. The overall mortality rate in older people with epilepsy remains 2–3 folds higher than general population of similar age group.[4]

Grown-ups with early-onset epilepsy is a characteristic subgroup as disparate from new-onset epilepsies in older people. This subgroup is different from older people with new-onset epilepsies in terms of etiological and risk factors, mortality, and morbidity risks and therapeutic considerations. We discuss some of the issues in the following text.

■ RISK AND ETIOLOGICAL FACTORS IN OLDER PEOPLE

Among very young people, the common etiological factors for epilepsy include, perinatal disorders, cortical developmental malformations, and central nervous system infections. In not so older people, the etiological spectrum changes to idiopathic epilepsies and traumatic brain injuries, and brain tumors. In older people, however, the common etiological factors responsible for epilepsy are distinctively different from younger age.

Cerebrovascular disease—ischemic and hemorrhagic combined is the most common etiology. Stroke accounts for nearly one-half of all new-onset epilepsies in the older age group. Ischemic strokes are major contributors to poststroke epilepsy series, given the higher incidence of ischemic in comparison to hemorrhagic strokes but the latter pose a higher risk of seizures as well as epilepsy. Seizures after stroke are categorized as early and late depending on whether they occur within 7 days after the cerebrovascular event or later. Early seizures are provoked or considered acute symptomatic. The risk of late seizures increases with middle cerebral artery strokes, cortical involvement, and higher severity of initial neurological insult. Calculating the SeLECT (severity of stroke, large-artery atherosclerotic etiology, early seizures, cortical involvement, territory of middle cerebral artery involvement) score which is formulated based on these risk factors, specifically after an ischemic stroke can aid in estimating the risk of remote symptomatic seizures.[5] Higher the score, more is the risk of seizure after the ischemic stroke. The risk of a late-unprovoked seizure is also elevated after an early seizure (<7 days) after stroke, but this does not mean that those people with early poststroke seizures on antiseizure medications (ASMs) in the long-term will reduce their risk of having late seizures in the long-term. The risk is especially greater in the first year following stroke but remains elevated for at least up to 10 years after stroke.

Seizures and epilepsy are common presenting manifestations as well as may occur later in the course of disease in many neurodegenerative conditions, in particular dementia of AD. It has been found that inheritance of *APOE4* mutation associates with subclinical epileptiform activity. Silent hippocampal seizures have been detected with intracranial foramen ovale electrodes in patients with AD. Also amnestic wandering in AD can be helped by ASM.[6] Other neurodegenerative disorders such as vascular dementia, Parkinson's disease, or other dementia conditions of old age also harbor a risk of increased risk of developing epilepsy as compared to general elderly population. The risk of epilepsy in elderly is especially higher in patients in which dementia and cerebrovascular disorders are present in the same individual. Traumatic brain injury poses a higher risk of epilepsy in elderly than it does in younger population. Physiological upset is much more common in older people and could result in acute symptomatic seizures, defined as seizure presenting with close temporal association with a brain insult.[7] Older persons are also prone to develop metabolic disturbances more commonly. Antihypertensives, diuretics, and antidepressants may lead to symptomatic hyponatremia in this age group. Though genetic generalized epilepsy is rare in these people, a relapse in people with history of (H/O) genetic epilepsy expected to be in long-term remission may occur with increasing life expectancy of these people. Notably, statin prescription, hypercholesterolemia, and an age older than 85 years are all independently associated with lower odds of developing epilepsy.[8]

■ EPILEPSY COMORBIDITIES IN OLDER PEOPLE

There is a complex interplay between comorbidities in older people with epilepsy. Optimizing patient care does require a holistic approach that not only targets seizure control but also all the domains affecting the activities of daily living of people growing old with epilepsy. The presence of comorbidities can still lead to a poor outcome in patients who have a very good seizure control from many years.

Cognition problems are of particular significance in older people with epilepsy. Apart from the age-related impairment in cognition, epilepsy itself is related to worsening of cognition overtime due to mechanisms unknown. It has been postulated that such progression of cognitive deficits might occur because of chronic accumulation of pathology (e.g., vascular) leading to epilepsy, effects of epilepsy itself (overt seizures or subclinical, abnormal cortical activity) or both.[9] Other researchers propose that an initial insult to the brain (e.g., stroke or traumatic brain injury) leads to cognitive function simply running below and parallel to the expected normal trajectory of cognitive change with aging[10] and that subsequent development of epilepsy is effectively a second hit, leading to even further deviation from expected decrement in cognition with aging.[11] Moreover, some ASMs contribute significantly to the cognitive decline. There is a bidirectional relationship between epilepsy and dementia, each increasing the risk of the occurrence of other. Reports suggest that cognitive decline might start several years earlier in people with mild cognitive impairment and AD who develop seizures compared with those who do not.[12] Epilepsy can be considered as one of the manifestations of underlying pathological process contributing to seizures, cognitive decline, systemic illness, psychological problems, etc.[10] One potential area of further research can be to establish that the processes leading to epileptogenesis can be modified through adjustment of vascular risk factors.

The older people with epilepsy also have a lot of psychosocial difficulties to tackle. The stigma of epilepsy, social isolation, effects on relationships, and dependency—all add on to the psychological burden affecting the quality of life they lead, making them prone to psychiatric comorbidities such as depression, anxiety, and sometimes psychosis. Though young people with epilepsy are much more prone to develop nonepileptic attacks, rare case reports of nonepileptic attacks in older adults with epilepsy are also present.

Age is the biggest risk factor for developing multimodal health difficulties. People with epilepsy are more likely to have additional somatic comorbidities such as musculoskeletal system disorders, respiratory system disorders, chronic pain disorders, diabetes, fractures, cerebrovascular accidents, etc., than general elderly population.[13]

Polypharmacy is most common in this age group, multiple drug interactions including the ASMs are to be considered while writing their prescriptions. Drug induced balance difficulties can increase risk of falls in them. Low bone density owing to the increasing age compounded by certain ASMs known to affect the bone health adversely can significantly increase the risk of pathological fractures in this age group. Getting a bone densitometry scan in older people with epilepsy thus becomes imperative. Various adverse effects of ASMs may lead the people taking them experience more debility than the seizure disorder itself, hence careful monitoring and regular follow-ups are strongly encouraged.

■ CLINICAL MANIFESTATIONS OF SEIZURES IN OLDER PEOPLE

Seizures in older people with epilepsy are distinctively different from seizures in younger people in terms of their clinical manifestations. Seizures in this age group may merely present with altered mental status, confusional episodes or wandering episodes, or just memory disturbance unlike the typical sensorimotor semiologies in the younger individuals. This makes it difficult to recognize seizures for emergency as well as other physicians. Both nonconvulsive seizures and status epilepticus (NCSE) are common among older individuals necessitating ambulatory continuous, long-term electroencephalographic (EEG) monitoring in those presenting with unexplained altered sensorium or lapses in sensorium. These features may last for several days and are sometimes preceding or followed by a bilateral tonic-clonic seizure. In the absence of EEG monitoring, NCSE may initially go unrecognized resulting in treatment delays.[14] In older people, auras are much less frequent, if at all present as generally nonspecific (e.g., dizziness), not allowing it to be of localizing value. Automatisms are likewise less frequent in older adults. On the contrary, postictal confusion can be considerably prolonged such that the older people with epilepsy can stay drowsy or confused up to days following a seizure episode and prolonged postictal hemiparesis in them may lead to misdiagnosis of a stroke.[15] EEG may not show typical epileptiform pattern in these older patients, hence diagnosis should be made based on both clinical and electrographic findings. Long-term and video-EEG are useful diagnostic tools in this population.[16] The differential diagnosis for epilepsy is broad in the elderly and includes syncope, metabolic disturbances, (e.g., hypoglycemia or hyperglycemia), transient ischemic attacks, cardiac events or arrhythmias, sleep disorders including REM-sleep behavior disorder, and psychogenic nonepileptic seizures, among other causes.[14]

Idiopathic Generalized Epilepsy in Older People

As a general rule, any new-onset epilepsy after the age of 25 years is focal unless proved otherwise. However, there are anecdotal reports of idiopathic generalized epilepsies manifesting for the first time in the adulthood and even in the seventh decade of life. On a different note, idiopathic generalized epilepsy, which is mostly acquired during adolescence affords better seizure control with advancing age. Contrary to the belief that many people with idiopathic generalized epilepsies, particularly juvenile myoclonic epilepsy require life-long treatment, there is a small proportion of people in their 40–50s, who experience seizure control even after coming off their ASMs.[15]

■ TREATMENT CONSIDERATIONS

New-onset epilepsy in older people is thought to be easily controlled with ASMs. This, however, does not mean that the management of epilepsy in older people is fairly uncomplicated. On a somewhat different note, the management of older people with early-onset epilepsy can be equally difficult having its own set of different challenges. To compound matters, there are very few controlled trials of the use of ASMs in older people with epilepsy.

The complexity of management of epilepsy in older people stems from a number of special considerations elaborated in the following text. Gastrointestinal absorption in older people is poor, slow, and often erratic. Serum albumin levels are often low in old age and this adversely impacts the serum concentrations of highly protein-bound ASMs, e.g., phenytoin, valproate, clobazam, and parempanel. There occurs a decline in the glomerular filtration rate and this impacts the plasma concentrations of several ASMs that are excreted via the kidney, e.g., levetiracetam, gabapentin, topiramate, and phenobarbital (of which 30% is excreted through the kidney). In addition, liver metabolizing enzyme capacity progressively diminishes along age and this will affect the metabolism of several ASMs that are metabolized in the liver, e.g., phenytoin, carbamazepine, valproate, lamotrigine, clobazam, and parempanel. Many, if not most older people with epilepsy, experience co- or multimorbidity and consequently are on polypharmacy. Many of their medications interact with ASMs through several mechanisms including the hepatic metabolizing enzymes (largely the cytochrome P-450 and the glucoronidation systems), displacement from protein binding, etc.

Special considerations are also due on account of declining bone health with advancing age, particularly in postmenopausal women, proclivity to falls, leading to injuries and fractures and a range of comorbidities. Several ASMs negatively impact bone health leading to osteoporosis through many different mechanisms reviewed elsewhere. These include hepatic P-450 enzyme-inducing ASMs such as phenobarbital, phenytoin, and carbamazepine but also noninducing ASMs like valproate. Older people with epilepsy also experience a range of psychiatric and somatic comorbidities, all of which are perhaps as common as among younger people with epilepsy. Two comorbidities stand out among the long list: cancer among somatic comorbidities and dementia among neurological comorbidities.

Clinical Trials of Antiseizure Medication in Older People

The Veteran's Affairs (VA) cooperative study randomized older people with epilepsy to either gabapentin 1,500 mg/day, lamotrigine 150 mg/day, or carbamazepine 600 mg/day. Retention rates were found better with lamotrigine in comparison to the other two medications.[16] The common side-effects in the trial included sedation, cognitive disturbances, gait disorders, and mood changes. In this trial as well as in clinical practice, it is the afore-mentioned list side-effects that lead to loss of retention of on ASM. Levetiracetam has similarly found to be safe and effective in older people with epilepsy. Of note, it was purported to improve selected but not all cognitive outcomes in a randomized trial of people with AD and epileptiform discharges on electroencephalography.[17] This particular property could be utilized to advantage in the treatment of epilepsy in older people with comorbid dementia.

The limited studies summarized in the earlier text inform us about choice of ASMs in older people with newly-diagnosed epilepsy. The choice, however, is also dictated by the range of comorbidities, comedications and their propensity to interact with ASMs, and contingent age-dependent physiological parameters involved in ASM kinetics. Some of the newer ASMs such as lamotrigine and levetiracetam offer benefits in terms of their favorable cognitive and bone health profiles, freedom from drug-drug interactions, and their demonstrated efficacy.

Lacosamide was well tolerated in the elderly aged 60 years and above, when given as add-on therapy for prolonged complex partial seizures, recurrent seizures, status epilepticus, and for chronic epilepsy over a mean follow-up period of 14 months. The mean daily dose of lacosamide was 368 mg (range: 100–600). The most frequent side effects were dizziness, fatigue, and tremor.[18]

Adjunctive brivaracetam was found to be efficacious, had good tolerability, and no new or unexpected side effects, when used to treat older patients with uncontrolled focal seizures in clinical practice as reported in the BRIVAFIRST (BRIVAracetam add-on First Italian netwoRk STudy) study.[19]

Treatment of Older People with Early-onset Epilepsy

Some people develop epilepsy at a young age and grow older with epilepsy and all along have been using ASMs. Many of them might be on older ASMs, which might have some of the limitations hitherto discussed. A proportion of them might continue to have seizures. In these people, it might be appropriate to switch to some of the newer ASMs, which have more favorable properties in regard to old age. In others, in whom, there is good seizure control, switching to alternative medications might be tricky.

Surgical Considerations

Till very recently, there was considerable nihilism for surgery for drug-resistant epilepsy in older people. This was largely based on the premise that age-related changes in brain networks and age and comorbidities might preclude a good surgical prognosis. However, recent experience from epilepsy surgical centers has shown that this is not the case and there is an increasing trend for older people to be admitted to surgical programs with outcomes nearly matching those in younger people.[20]

■ CONCLUSION

Epilepsy in elderly is a cause of growing concern given the increasing quanta of people falling into this category which is expected to grow further in near future. Older people differ significantly than other age groups in clinical presentation of seizures, etiology of epilepsy, pharmacokinetics, co-morbid profile and response to antiseizure medications—mandating special considerations for this age group. Surgical consideration in these people is also gaining importance and surgical outcome has been shown to be comparable with the younger people.

REFERENCES

1. Beghi E, Giussani G, Costa C, DiFrancesco JC, Dhakar M, Leppik I, et al. The epidemiology of epilepsy in older adults: A narrative review by the ILAE Task Force on Epilepsy in the Elderly. Epilepsia. 2023;64(3):586-601.
2. GBD 2016 Epilepsy Collaborators. Global, regional, and national burden of epilepsy, 1990-2016: a systematic analysis for the Global Burden of Disease Study 2016. Lancet Neurol. 2019;18(4):357-75.
3. Sillanpää M, Gissler M, Schmidt D. Efforts in Epilepsy Prevention in the Last 40 Years: Lessons From a Large Nationwide Study. JAMA Neurol. 2016;73(4):390-5.
4. Lhatoo SD, Johnson AL, Goodridge DM, MacDonald BK, Sander JW, Shorvon SD. Mortality in epilepsy in the first 11 to 14 years after diagnosis: multivariate analysis of a long-term, prospective, population-based cohort. Ann Neurol. 2001;49(3):336-44.
5. Galovic M, Döhler N, Erdélyi-Canavese B, Felbecker A, Siebel P, Conrad J, et al. Prediction of late seizures after ischaemic stroke with a novel prognostic model (the SeLECT score): a multivariable prediction model development and validation study. Lancet Neurol. 2018;17(2):143-52.
6. Vossel KA, Ranasinghe KG, Beagle AJ, Mizuiri D, Honma SM, Dowling AF, et al. Incidence and impact of subclinical epileptiform activity in Alzheimer's disease. Ann Neurol. 2016;80(6):858-70.
7. Beghi E, Carpio A, Forsgren L, Hesdorffer DC, Malmgren K, Sander JW, et al. Recommendation for a definition of acute symptomatic seizure. Epilepsia. 2010;51(4):671-5.
8. Pugh MJ, Knoefel JE, Mortensen EM, Amuan ME, Berlowitz DR, Van Cott AC. New-onset epilepsy risk factors in older veterans. J Am Geriatr Soc. 2009;57(2):237-42.
9. Seidenberg M, Pulsipher DT, Hermann B. Cognitive progression in epilepsy. Neuropsychol Rev. 2007;17(4):445-54.
10. Helmstaedter C, Elger CE. Chronic temporal lobe epilepsy: a neurodevelopmental or progressively dementing disease? Brain. 2009;132(Pt 10):2822-30.
11. Sen A, Capelli V, Husain M. Cognition and dementia in older patients with epilepsy. Brain. 2018;141(6):1592-608.
12. Pandis D, Scarmeas N. Seizures in Alzheimer disease: clinical and epidemiological data. Epilepsy Curr. 2012;12(5):184-7.

13. Seidenberg M, Pulsipher DT, Hermann B. Association of Epilepsy and Comorbid Conditions. Future Neurology. 2009;4(5):663-8.
14. Sarkis RA, Schrettner M. Seizures and Epilepsy in the Elderly.-Practical Neurology. [online] Available from https://practicalneurology.com/articles/2018-mar-apr/seizures-and-epilepsy-in-the-elderly [Last accessed September, 2024].
15. Janz D. Epilepsy with impulsive petit mal (juvenile myoclonic epilepsy). Acta Neurol Scand. 1985;72(5):449-59.
16. Rowan AJ, Ramsay RE, Collins JF, Pryor F, Boardman KD, Uthman BM, et al; VA Cooperative Study 428 Group. New onset geriatric epilepsy: a randomized study of gabapentin, lamotrigine, and carbamazepine. Neurology. 2005;64(11):1868-73.
17. Vossel K, Ranasinghe KG, Beagle AJ, La A, Ah Pook K, Castro M, et al. Effect of Levetiracetam on Cognition in Patients With Alzheimer Disease With and Without Epileptiform Activity: A Randomized Clinical Trial. JAMA Neurol. 2021;78(11):1345-54.
18. Rainesalo S, Mäkinen J, Raitanen J, Peltola J. Clinical management of elderly patients with epilepsy; the use of lacosamide in a single center setting. Epilepsy Behav. 2017;75:86-9.
19. Lattanzi S, Canafoglia L, Canevini MP, Casciato S, Cerulli Irelli E, Chiesa V, et al.; BRIVAFIRST Group Membership. Adjunctive Brivaracetam in Older Patients with Focal Seizures: Evidence from the BRIVAracetam add on First Italian netwoRk Study (BRIVAFIRST). Drugs Aging. 2022;39(4):297-304.
20. Punia V, Sheikh SR, Thompson NR, Bingaman W, Jehi L. Quality of life before and after epilepsy surgery: Age is just a number. Epilepsy Behav. 2020;113:107574.

Management of Women with Epilepsy

Parthvi Shreyas Ravat, Aditya Sunil Gudhate, Sangeeta Ravat

ABSTRACT

This review provides an overview of the complexities involved in managing epilepsy in women across various life stages. It emphasizes the importance of a multifaceted approach that addresses not only seizure control but also hormonal fluctuations, pregnancy considerations, fertility, bone health, and psychological well-being.

Key considerations are hormonal influences and contraception necessitating individualized treatment plans. Effective contraception is critical for women with epilepsy (WWE) due to the heightened risk of unplanned pregnancies and potential complications. Enzyme-inducing antiseizure medications (ASMs) can interact with hormonal contraceptives, making intrauterine devices (IUDs) the preferred choice for contraception in this population. Seizure control during pregnancy is discussed. Dosage adjustments of most ASMs are necessary to maintain efficacy and require neurologists to be familiar with latest research. Preconception counseling is highly recommended to optimize seizure control and fetal outcomes. Breastfeeding is encouraged for WWE with most ASMs being compatible with it, with minimal risks of adverse effects on the infant. However, monitoring may be needed for infants exposed to specific ASMs. Concerns exist regarding congenital malformations, prematurity, and developmental deficits in the offspring. Risk profiles of different drugs and prevention strategies are discussed. Special populations such as elderly women, women with osteoporosis and psychiatric comorbidities, sexual dysfunction and their particular concerns are addressed with latest available research, emphasizing a multi-disciplinary approach for comprehensive care.

Keywords: Epilepsy, Reproductive medicine, Menopause, Contraception and epilepsy, Antiseizure medicine.

■ CLINICAL SCENARIO

A 29-year-old woman with refractory idiopathic generalized epilepsy wishes to conceive. She has been trialed on multiple antiseizure medications (ASM), including levetiracetam (LEV), lamotrigine (LTG), topiramate (TOP), carbamazepine (CBZ), and oxcarbazepine (OxCBZ), at appropriate dosages and for adequate duration, but her seizures remain controlled only with valproate (VPA) at a dose of 500 mg twice a day. Her current valproate total and free serum levels are in the upper therapeutic range. Lower doses of valproate had never been tried.

Question: How do you advise her regarding ASM and pregnancy, risks to the fetus, and risks of her having seizures?

Patient trajectory: Over 6 months, her VPA dosage was reduced to 200 mg twice daily, but she experienced a recurrent generalized tonic–clonic seizure. Maintaining VPA at 200 mg twice daily, LEV 500 mg twice daily was added and well-tolerated. She received a detailed counseling about the risks of major congenital malformations (MCMs) and cognitive-behavioral outcomes associated with VPA. She was also told about the minimal neurodevelopmental effects of LEV on the offspring such as anxiety. After 9 months of seizure freedom, she naturally conceived and, with close monitoring, delivered a healthy, full-term baby girl.

■ LEARNING POINTS

This case underscores the complexities of managing women with epilepsy (WWE) who want to conceive and are not well-controlled on almost all ASMs except VPA. VPA should be avoided in all people with epilepsy of childbearing potential (PWECP), if possible. However, a small proportion of women, especially those with idiopathic generalized epilepsy, may only achieve optimal seizure control with VPA. If monotherapy with alternative medications fails or the patient declines changes after detailed preconception counseling, reconsidering VPA at the lowest effective dose should be considered, guided by serum drug levels. The lowest effective dose must be individualized and reevaluated over time. Discovering an unintended pregnancy long after neural tube closure is not uncommon since over 50% of WWE have unplanned pregnancies, many with delayed recognition. However, it is to be noted that when monotherapy trials fail, polytherapy with low-dose VPA may pose a lower risk than high-dose VPA monotherapy. If there is a history of prior abortions, miscarriages, or neural tube defects in the offspring, it further increases the risk of having MCMs. Thus, coprescribing high-dose folic acid combined with early fetal assessment best ensured her desired pregnancy outcome.

■ INTRODUCTION

Epilepsy is a chronic disorder in the majority of patients and requires long-term management during various phases of life. In women with epilepsy (WWE) the hormonal military is changing from adolescence and puberty—menarche and menstruation, pregnancy, breastfeeding, and then menopause. It is important to address epilepsy-related concerns at each stage. Epilepsy management involves a comprehensive approach beyond simply controlling seizures. This includes addressing psychiatric issues, metabolic- and endocrine- related issues (bone, thyroid, etc.), social stigma and ways to deal with it, cognitive clouding, and many more in WWE.

■ HORMONAL INFLUENCES

Catamenial Epilepsy

Catamenial is derived from the Greek work "katamenios", which means monthly, and narrates a seizure pattern that correlates with the 4 phases of the menstrual cycle: Menstrual, follicular, ovulatory, and luteal. Catamenia epilepsy (CE) is defined as the doubling of seizures or seizures occurring almost exclusively during specific times of the menstrual cycle. This is to be noted more specifically during the following phases: Perimenstrual (catamenial pattern 1—C1), periovulatory (catamenial pattern 2—C2), and luteal (catamenial pattern 3—C3) in anovulatory cycle.[1] Extensive seizure and menstrual history help in developing a correlation between the two, and thus arriving at the diagnosis. Patients must be taught how to maintain a seizure diary along with a period/menstrual tracker. The utility of daily tracking tools plays an important role in accurate ascertainment of CE, especially when considering personalized treatment approaches.[2]

The treatment options depend on the regularity of the menstrual cycle. For females with regular menstrual cycles (C1 and C2) and who can be expected to track their cycles and seizures well, hormonal and nonhormonal treatments can be offered.

Hormonal therapy is pulsed in the second half of the menstrual cycle (day 14–15 to day 25–28) in varying doses (600 mg/day[3] or 80 mg/day[4]). This has shown some changes in mean seizure frequency (moderate-to-low, certainty evidence of no treatment difference between progesterone and placebo) but clubbed with side effects like menstrual irregularities and headaches in these females.[1,3,4] The efficacy of pulsed progesterone is yet to be seen in large randomized control trial.[5] Other investigational hormonal therapies include ganaxolone, clomiphene citrate, and natural progesterone lozenges.[6]

Nonhormonal treatments include clobazam or acetazolamide, which can be taken prior to and during the 5–7 days of ongoing menstrual bleeding. Clobazam, a benzodiazepine, is known to reduce seizures in the majority of CE patients[7] and the monthly cyclical dosing helps prevent the expected benzodiazepine tolerance. Acetazolamide, a carbonic anhydrase inhibitor, has poor literature to support its usage but has been historically used in refractory epilepsies for seizure control. It has been tried in cyclical dosage (C1 and C2 patterns) and in daily dosing regimen in the C3 pattern of CE.[8,9]

In women with irregular menstruation (C3), a complete cessation of menstruation using synthetic hormones (e.g. medroxyprogesterone (Depo-Provera) or gonadotropin-releasing hormone (GnRH) analogs (triptorelin and goserelin) should be considered to achieve seizure control.[1]

Contraception

A majority (up to 60%) of the pregnancies in the general population are unplanned, and these unplanned pregnancies double the risk of spontaneous fetal loss in WWE.[10] They might also be associated with increased rates of premature delivery, low birth weight, congenital anomalies, and infant mortality.[11,12] Intermenstrual bleeding is an indicator of contraceptive failure, but does not always occur. The reasons for unplanned pregnancy are myriad. They can range from not using highly effective contraception methods such as barrier, withdrawal, or combinations of those; or using hormonal contraception while on an enzyme-inducing antiseizure medication (ASM), thus posing a risk of contraceptive failure.[13,10] Thus, the importance of effective contraception in WWE is very high.

However, the relationship between contraceptives and ASM is complicated. This bidirectional relationship is shown in **Flowchart 1**. Many enzyme-inducing agents are known to reduce the levels of ASMs, and thus increase seizure risk. The most commonly used current oral hormonal contraceptives contain 20–35 µg of ethinyl estradiol and <1 mg of progesterone. The World Health Organization (WHO) advises against using combined oral contraceptive pills (COCP), the vaginal ring, and the transdermal patch while on enzyme-inducing ASM.[14] If one must use an oral method of contraception, then a high-dose preparation containing at least 50 µg or more of the estrogen compound is recommended. Besides their effect on contraceptives, enzyme-inducing ASMs lower serum levels of folates, and enzyme inhibitor such as valproate (VPA) acts as a folate antagonist.[15]

When it comes to the effect of contraceptives on ASMs, estrogen, especially the ethinyl estradiol part is known to reduce the concentrations of VPA and lamotrigine (LTG),

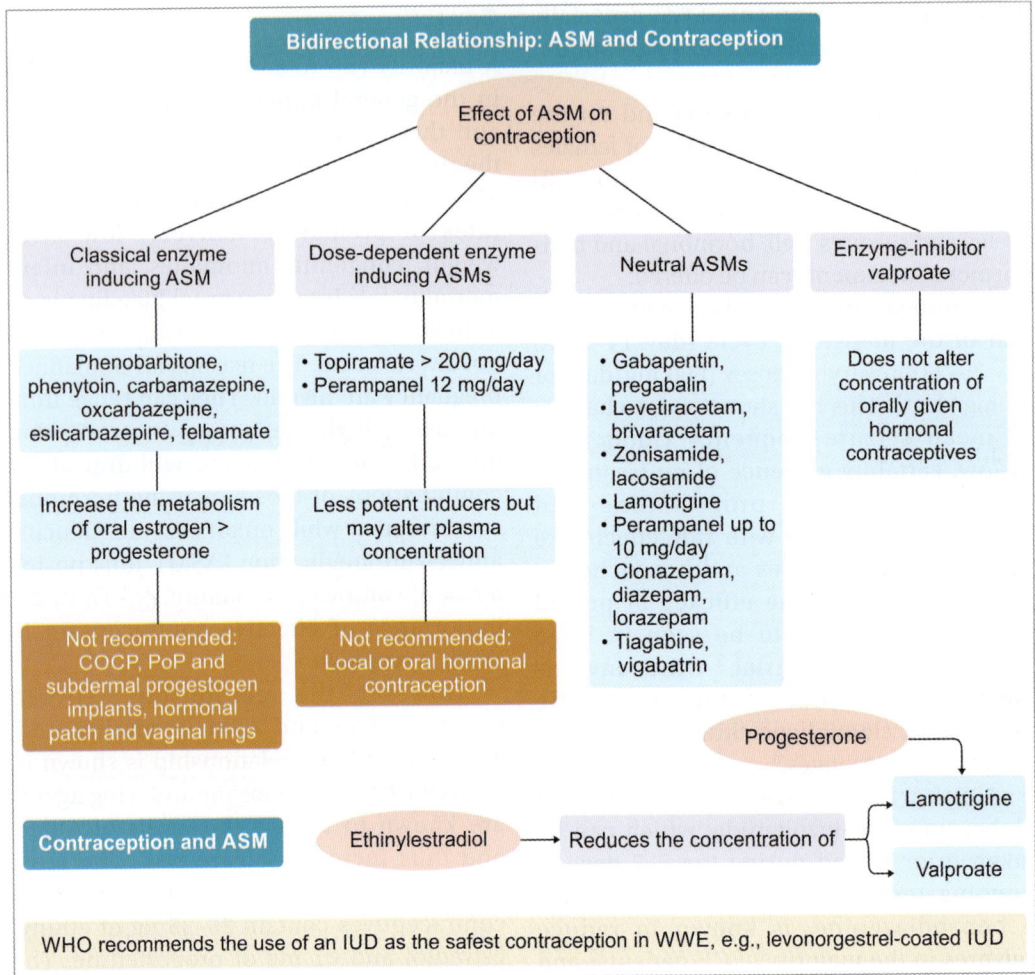

FLOWCHART 1: Balancing ASM and contraception.
(ASM: antiseizure medication; COCP: combined oral contraceptive pills; IUD: intrauterine device; PoP: progestogen-only pill; WHO: World Health Organization; WWE: women without epilepsy)

possibly by the mechanism of accelerated glucuronidation.[16-18] This leads to loss of seizure control in WWE, taking both COCP and LTG. Progesterone has also been noted to reduce the levels of LTG.

This understanding of interactions between ASM and contraceptives can aid in optimizing therapy for WWE before there is a breakthrough seizure or failure of contraception **(Flowchart 1)**. Depot medroxyprogesterone acetate (MPA) injections are effective for all ASM categories, but they have significant side effects, which make them a less favorable option, such as constant vaginal bleeding[19], weight gain[19], delayed return to fertility, and impaired bone health.[20] WHO, thus, recommends the use of intrauterine devices (IUD) as a first choice of contraception in the majority of WWE, with the advantage of no relevant drug–drug interactions. This can be a classical IUD, copper-coated IUD, or the newer levonorgestrel-releasing IUD. The levonorgestrel IUD appears to be effective, even in women taking enzyme-inducing ASMs and seems as well-tolerated in WWE than in women without epilepsy.

Neutral ASMs: Available data, although sparse, suggest that gabapentin, pregabalin, LEV, brivaracetam, zonisamide, and lacosamide do not affect the metabolism of oral contraceptives. Perampanel up to 10 mg/day also appears safe. These may be preferred in WWE.

Contraceptive counseling by epileptologists and specific mention of an IUD are significantly associated with patient's selection of an IUD as a contraceptive method, thus emphasizing how important is the role of a neurologist in patients' contraceptive choices and, thus, seizure management.[21]

Thyroid Disorders

Regular monitoring of thyroid function, including thyroid-stimulating hormone (TSH), free thyroxine (FT4), and thyroid peroxidase antibodies (TPOAb) levels, is crucial for early detection of thyroid dysfunction in women with epilepsy.[22,23] Choosing the right ASM in people with epilepsy of childbearing potential (PWECP) with already diagnosed thyroid disorders can help avert complications. Phenytoin, CBZ, and phenobarbital lead to increased clearance of thyroxine (T4) and have a potential for subclinical hypothyroidism, even with normal TSH levels.[24] LEV has minimal to no effect on thyroid function, while the evidence for LTG is less clear.[25]

■ PREGNANCY

Seizure control is vital during the 40 weeks of gestational period. Convulsive seizures can lead to blunt trauma, lactic acidosis,[26] and ictal hypoxia in both the mother and fetus.[27] Convulsive status epilepticus can have far worse consequences than those of brief seizures. In women with previously well-controlled epilepsy, the pregnancy is usually uneventful. Most ASMs (e.g., LTG, OxCBZe, and LEV) need to be increased to compensate for the decline in serum levels; exceptions are VPA and CBZ.[26] Therapeutic drug monitoring should begin early in pregnancy, and increasing doses of these anticonvulsants may be needed throughout the course of pregnancy.[28]

There is no significant difference found in the mode of delivery in WWE and pregnant controls. However, unlabored/elective cesarean rates are higher among WWE irrespective of type and dosage of ASM. Provider preference may influence delivery mode among WWE as this was found in community hospitals only and not in tertiary care hospitals.[29]

Preconception Checklist

Preconceptional counseling is arguably the most important information a WWE receives in order to minimize the teratogenic risk of ASMs and optimize seizure control prior to getting pregnant. It is very important to have a joint decision-making system between the neurologist and the patient in order to optimize both seizure control and fetal outcomes.[30] Recently, released guidelines by the American Academy of Neurology for PWECP have been summarized in a graphical summary by the Young Epilepsy Section of International League Against Epilepsy, which can be found here https://www.ilae.org/education/infographics#Teratogenesis. WWE should be reassured that the majority of pregnancies are uneventful.

Folic Acid

Neural tube closure occurs within the first 28 days after conception. The most common congenital malformations are neural tube defects (NTD) characterized by incomplete closure of the embryonic neural tube, including anencephaly and spina bifida.[31] Low levels of maternal folate can be a causative factor for this.[32] Some ASMs, especially VPA (folate antagonist) and CBZ have been shown to cause NTDs. Many studies have shown that periconceptional folic acid supplementation cannot reduce ASM-associated malformations[33,34] and have no overall effect on women on ASM during pregnancy.[35,36] However, it may have a protective effect against fetal ASM-induced language delay and autistic traits, and also might lead to a higher intelligence quotient (IQ) level.[37-39] NTDs occur during the first 4 weeks of pregnancy, between 21 and 28 days after conception, when most women are unaware of their pregnancies, supporting the need for folate supplementation as a preconception intervention.

More randomized control trials would be the ideal way to study the appropriate folate dosage. However, all WWE should be encouraged to continue ASM as well as supplement folic acid with 0.4–0.8 mg/day before and while pregnant.[40] This will decrease the risk of NTDs in the offspring (Level B)[30] and possibly improve neurodevelopmental outcomes such as autism spectrum disorder (ASD) and global IQ in the offspring (Level A).

Postpartum Care

Breastfeeding is extremely important for the baby's nutrition and should begin within 1 hour of birth. Widely recognized negative effects of specific ASMs on fetal development are not the same during the breastfeeding period.

Women with epilepsy who are not on ASM can breastfeed without any concerns. For WWE who are on ASMs, recent data[41] supports the breastfeeding of infants. This is mainly because ASM concentration in blood samples of breastfed newborns was substantially lower than maternal blood concentration. Exposure to ASMs via breastmilk does not cause clinically significant adverse effects for the majority of breastfed infants.[42] The benefits of breastfeeding versus the risks of ASM to the baby need to be assessed on an individual case basis. Most of the ASMs, including LTG, LEV, CBZ, TOP, VPA, and gabapentin, do not produce significant adverse effects that would warrant discontinuing breastfeeding. These ASMs did not seem to retard the growth, development, IQ, and verbal abilities of the breastfed infants.[43-45]

However, infants exposed to phenobarbital, primidone, and these ASMs via breast milk might be monitored for signs of poor suckling/inadequate weight gain, sedation/drowsiness/irritability, iLTG via breast milk might warrant monitoring for apnea and rashes [46] It has been recommended that breastfeeding be limited or discontinued in case of excessive sedation/drowsiness and/or poor weight gain.[43] Accumulation of ASM in the infant can occur, especially with high breast milk levels in ASMs such as LEV or LTG. However, breastfed infants had very low LEV serum concentrations, suggesting a rapid elimination of LEV.[47] Fetal hepatotoxicity has also been seen in breastfed babies of mothers taking VPA. One strategy to tackle this is to avoid breastfeeding during periods of peak maternal plasma drug concentration.

In the mothers, postpartum baseline levels of ASM are reached relatively fast, and down-titration is performed empirically[26] WWE should never stop medication abruptly, as she may have seizures, and the baby may also experience drug withdrawal.

The general expert opinion is that WWE, taking ASMs, should be encouraged to breastfeed, just like the general population. This is based on the assumption that the manifold advantages of breast milk outweigh any harm from a modest drug exposure.[48]

MANAGEMENT AND RISKS TO OFFSPRINGS

The majority of the births in WWE are normal. The risk to mothers and babies is small and preventable. Nonetheless, some concerns exist about birth defects such as NTDs and malformations, small gestational age babies (SGA), and developmental deficits while growing up.

Major Congenital Malformations

The overall malformation risk in the general population is 2.4–2.9%. LTG (3.1%), LEV (3.5%), and OxCBZ (3.1%) are associated with the lowest risk of MCMs, similar to the general population. VPA was associated with the highest risk of MCM (9.7%)—NTDs and urogenital and renal malformations. TOP is associated with SGA. Polytherapy with VPA and any other ASM is highly teratogenic and appears to be even worse in combination with LTG (1 of 10 infants exposed). Hence, it is a reasonable practice to use the lowest appropriate dose of ASMs in PWECP, if clinically feasible[30] and avoid VPA altogether. Pregnancy registries are helpful, and doctors can access them to find an update about data related to any particular ASM. A large Indian pregnancy registry is the Kerala (India) Registry of Epilepsy and Pregnancy, established in 1998, and one must encourage Indian pregnant patients to enroll in these registries to aid research, and thus improve patient care.

Neurodevelopmental Outcomes

Valproate and TOP use during pregnancy is associated with a significantly increased risk of neurodevelopmental effects on the fetus.[49] VPA is linked to a significant risk of developing ASD,[50-52] attention-deficit/hyperactivity disorder (ADHD), impaired cognitive function, intellectual disability, and attachment disorder in the offspring but no association was found with a risk of later-onset psychiatric disorders, such as anxiety, mood disorders, substance use, or schizophrenia spectrum disorders.[53] LEV, a commonly used drug in pregnancy, has significantly increased rates of ADHD diagnosis and anxiety in the offspring over a long-term follow-up.[53] The data for other ASMs is scant. However, LTG seems free of adverse neurodevelopmental effects.[49]

Screening guidelines during pregnancy involve ultrasound scans in every trimester, anomaly scan at 18 weeks, serum alpha-fetoprotein, and karyotyping during pregnancy. In case an abnormality is found in the fetus on one of these screens, the Indian constitution allows the right of abortion of the fetus to the mother up to 20 weeks of gestation. Almost all NTDs can be detected by 20 weeks.

Genetic testing in WWE can be encouraged for precision medicine, prognosis, family planning, possible future therapies, and a reduction of iatrogeny.[54] But not all genetic causes of epilepsy are known, and a negative test does not rule out a genetic cause. Furthermore, the discovery of a genetic mutation can have psychological impacts on the individual and their family.

SPECIAL POPULATIONS

Young Women

Idiopathic Generalized Epilepsies in Females

The most common idiopathic generalized epilepsies (IGE) syndrome is juvenile myoclonic epilepsy, with a marked female predominance.[55] VPA is the conventional drug of choice.[56,57] Considering a heavy side effect profile, high rates of congenital malformations, and poor neurodevelopmental outcomes in the offspring, VPA must not be used in PWECP. In planning a switch, there is evidence for a reduced risk of recurrence or worsening with LEV as compared to LTG.[58] Factors involved in predicting a high risk of recurrence include high preexisting VPA dosage, multiple seizure types, shorter remission times from generalized tonic–clonic seizure (GTCS), and catamenial worsening of seizures.[58] In case of poor control, rational polytherapy is considered better than VPA for PWECP.

Fertility

Birth rates among WWE are lower than in the general population.[59] This is not the same for fertility rates. WWE has similar chances of achieving pregnancy, time to pregnancy, and live birth rates compared to controls.[60] Fertility is independent of birth rates as WWE might choose not to get pregnant despite being fertile for various other reasons such as difficulty finding a partner, social stigma associated with epilepsy, and difficulty in raising a child when one has epilepsy.

There is an increased risk of infertility in women taking three or more different ASMs compared with WWE not taking medication.[61] However, therapy with ASM did not decrease the chance of live birth in women in the cohort of WWE who underwent assisted reproduction.[62] The chances of a live birth per embryo transfer were similar in WWE and controls.[62] These are encouraging findings for WWE and helpful to the physician/obstetrician while counseling WWE regarding an assisted pregnancy.

Elderly Women

Menopause

There is varying evidence for a fluctuation of seizure frequency and severity during menopause.[63] Menopause can be accompanied by mood changes, anxiety, and depression, which can potentially exacerbate epilepsy. Optimizing seizure control with the least-risky medication options is essential.

TABLE 1: Hormone replacement therapy (HRT): Risks and benefits.

Potential benefits	Potential risks
Management of menopausal symptoms like hot flashes, night sweats, and vaginal dryness	Increased risk of breast cancer
Decreased seizure frequency in certain women with epilepsy (WWE)[65]	Increased risk of blood clots
Women with well-controlled epilepsy may be more likely to benefit from HRT compared to those with uncontrolled seizures. Addition of natural progesterone may reduce effects of estrogen-related seizure frequency rise[66]	Potential for interactions with antiseizure medications
	Catamenial epilepsy might be more influenced by hormonal changes

Source: Adapted from Harden et al. (2006).

A study comparing the effects of LTG and LEV suggests a potential advantage over traditional ASM as they do not affect bone density.[64] The exact role of hormone replacement therapy (HRT) in WWE is not clear but potential risks and benefits are enumerated in **Table 1**.

Bone Health

Serum vitamin D levels should be measured before the initiation of treatment and then at 6–12 months with enzyme-inducing ASMs. The National Institute for Clinical Excellence (NICE, 2017) recommends the tests of bone metabolism every 2–5 years for adults taking enzyme-inducing ASMs. The frequency of monitoring depends on individual risk factors and bone mineral density (BMD) results. The National Osteoporosis Foundation recommends repeating dual-energy X-ray absorptiometry (DXA) scans every 2–3 years for low bone mass (T-score of –1.0 to –2.5) and every 1–2 years for osteoporosis (T-score below –2.5). For WWE, especially those on enzyme-inducing ASMs or with additional risk factors, more frequent monitoring (e.g., every 1–2 years) may be warranted. In severe cases of osteoporosis, bisphosphonate therapy may be considered to increase bone mineral density and reduce fracture risk.[67,68] Lifestyle modifications in the form of weight-bearing exercise and a healthy diet rich in calcium and vitamin D can significantly improve bone health. Exposure to sunlight which is shown to be beneficial for bone health must be encouraged as many patients with refractory epilepsy often do not leave their house due to fear of seizures.

PSYCHOSOCIAL ASPECTS IN WOMEN WITH EPILEPSY

Social implications including concerns about societal stigma, disclosure of diagnosis, and anxiety associated with this can lead to a delay in marriage or create marital strain. Studies in India, for instance, reveal a reluctance to disclose epilepsy before marriage, impacting trust and marital satisfaction.[69]

The coexistence of psychogenic non-epileptic seizures (PNES) also complicates epilepsy management, which has a higher prevalence rate in WWE as compared to males with epilepsy.[70] PNES occurs in the mid-to-late twenties, the disorder can affect individuals across all age groups with higher incidence in females.[71] This is perhaps due to greater psychiatric comorbidity and social stigma in this population. Treatment includes a multidimensional approach with cognitive behavioral therapy and antidepressants.

The WWE experience higher rates of sexual dysfunction compared to the general population, which can manifest as decreased desire, arousal difficulties, problems with lubrication, and orgasmic dysfunction.[72] Strategies to promote sexual well-being can start with open communication with partners about epilepsy and the desired support. Addressing underlying anxiety or depression through therapy can positively impact sexual function.[73]

Women with epilepsy also are more likely to develop depression;[74] anxiety disorders, including generalized anxiety disorder and social anxiety disorder;[75] post-traumatic stress disorder (PTSD); and bipolar disorder.[76] ASMs, particularly enzyme-inducing medications (e.g., phenytoin, CBZ, and phenobarbital), can increase the metabolism of antidepressants and antipsychotics, leading to decreased blood levels and potentially reduced therapeutic effects.[77] Newer ASMs like LTG and LEV have minimal enzyme-inducing effects and pose less risk for pharmacokinetic interactions.[77] Selective serotonin reuptake inhibitors (SSRIs) like fluoxetine and sertraline are generally considered safe for use with ASMs, while tricyclic antidepressants (TCAs) may have more interaction potential.[78] Typical antipsychotics (second-generation) are generally preferred due to a lower risk of seizure threshold lowering compared to typical antipsychotics (first-generation).[79] Monitoring blood levels of ASMs and coadministered medications like antidepressants or antipsychotics can be helpful to ensure optimal therapeutic effects and minimize the risk of adverse reactions.

FUTURE DIRECTIVES

To address the pressing needs in epilepsy research for PWECP, several critical areas must be prioritized. First, there is a need to study newer ASMs, such as lacosamide, zonisamide, clobazam, cenobamate, perampanel, and fenfluramine, to determine their safety and efficacy in this population. Neurodevelopmental outcomes and their relation to dosages of ASM and dosage of folic acid are another areas requiring research, inclusive of diverse ethnic and racial groups, people from low- and middle-income countries, as well as transgender, nonbinary, and intersex PWECP, to ensure that findings are applicable to all affected populations.

CONCLUSION

Our review emphasizes the need to study newer ASMs, to determine their safety and efficacy in this population. Neurodevelopmental outcomes and their relation to dosages of ASM, dosage of folic acid is another area requiring research, inclusive of diverse ethnic and racial groups, people from low and middle-income countries, as well as transgender, nonbinary, and intersex PWECP, to ensure that findings are applicable to all affected populations.

REFERENCES

1. Maguire MJ, Nevitt SJ. Treatments for seizures in catamenial (menstrual-related) epilepsy. Cochrane Database Syst Rev. 2019;2019(10):CD013225.
2. Voinescu PE, Kelly M, French JA, Harden C, Davis A, Lau C, et al. Catamenial epilepsy occurrence and patterns in a mixed population of women with epilepsy. Epilepsia. 2023;64(9):e194-9.
3. Herzog AG, Fowler KM, Smithson SD, Kalayjian LA, Heck CN, Sperling MR, et al.; Progesterone Trial Study Group. Progesterone vs placebo therapy for women with epilepsy: A randomized clinical trial. Neurology. 2012;78(24):1959-66.
4. Najafi M, Sadeghi MM, Mehvari J, Zare M, Akbari M. Progesterone therapy in women with intractable catamenial epilepsy. Adv Biomed Res. 2013;2:8.
5. Nucera B, Rinaldi F, Dono F, Lanzone J, Evangelista G, Consoli S, et al. Progesterone and its derivatives for the treatment of catamenial epilepsy: A systematic review. Seizure. 2023;109:52-9.
6. Practical Neurology. (2022). Catamenial epilepsy. [online]. Available from https://practicalneurology.com/articles/2022-oct/catamenial-epilepsy. [Last accessed September, 2024].
7. Feely M, Calvert R, Gibson J. Clobazam in catamenial epilepsy. A model for evaluating anticonvulsants. Lancet. 1982;2(8289):71-3.
8. Lim LL, Foldvary N, Mascha E, Lee J. Acetazolamide in women with catamenial epilepsy. Epilepsia. 2001;42(6):746-9.
9. Turner AL, Perry MS. Outside the box: Medications worth considering when traditional antiepileptic drugs have failed. Seizure. 2017;50:173-85.
10. Herzog AG, Mandle HB, MacEachern DB. Association of unintended pregnancy with spontaneous fetal loss in women with epilepsy. JAMA Neurol. 2019;76(1):50-5.
11. Orr ST, Miller CA, James SA, Babones S. Unintended pregnancy and preterm birth. Paediatr Perinat Epidemiol. 2000;14(4):309-13.
12. Mohllajee AP, Curtis KM, Morrow B, Marchbanks PA. Pregnancy intention and its relationship to birth and maternal outcomes. Obstet Gynecol. 2007;109(3):678-86.
13. Herzog AG, Mandle HB, MacEachern DB. Prevalence of highly effective contraception use by women with epilepsy. Neurology. 2019;92(24):e2815-21.
14. Gaffield ME, Culwell KR, Lee CR. The use of hormonal contraception among women taking anticonvulsant therapy. Contraception. 2011;83(1):16-29.
15. Herzog AG, MacEachern DB, Mandle HB, Cahill KE, Fowler KM, Davis AR, et al. Folic acid use by women with epilepsy: Findings of the Epilepsy Birth Control Registry. Epilepsy Behav. 2017;72:156-60.
16. Sabers A, Buchholt JM, Uldall P, Hansen EL. Lamotrigine plasma levels reduced by oral contraceptives. Epilepsy Res. 2001;47(1-2):151-4.
17. Galimberti CA, Mazzucchelli I, Arbasino C, Canevini MP, Fattore C, Perucca E. Increased apparent oral clearance of valproic acid during intake of combined contraceptive steroids in women with epilepsy. Epilepsia. 2006;47(9):1569-72.
18. Herzog AG, Blum AS, Farina EL, Maestri XE, Newman J, Garcia E, et al. Valproate and

lamotrigine level variation with menstrual cycle phase and oral contraceptive use. Neurology. 2009;72(10):911-4.
19. Archer B, Irwin D, Jensen K, Johnson ME, Rorie J. Depot medroxyprogesterone. Management of side-effects commonly associated with its contraceptive use. J Nurse Midwifery. 1997;42(2):104-11.
20. Dupont S, Vercueil L. Epilepsy and pregnancy: What should the neurologists do? Rev Neurol (Paris). 2021;177(3):168-79.
21. Espinera AR, Gavvala J, Bellinski I, Kennedy J, Macken MP, Narechania A, et al. Counseling by epileptologists affects contraceptive choices of women with epilepsy. Epilepsy Behav. 2016;65:1-6.
22. Tamijani SM, Karimi B, Amini E, Golpich M, Dargahi L, Ali RA, et al. Thyroid hormones: Possible roles in epilepsy pathology. Seizure. 2015;31:155-64.
23. Weatherburn CJ, Heath CA, Mercer SW, Guthrie B. Physical and mental health comorbidities of epilepsy: Population-based cross-sectional analysis of 1.5 million people in Scotland. Seizure. 2017;45:125-31.
24. Han Y, Yang J, Zhong R, Guo X, Cai M, Lin W. Side effects of long-term oral anti-seizure drugs on thyroid hormones in patients with epilepsy: A systematic review and network meta-analysis. Neurol Sci. 2022;43(9):5217-27.
25. Rochtus AM, Herijgers D, Jansen K, Decallonne B. Antiseizure medications and thyroid hormone homeostasis: Literature review and practical recommendations. Epilepsia. 2022;63(2):259-70.
26. Nucera B, Brigo F, Trinka E, Kalss G. Treatment and care of women with epilepsy before, during, and after pregnancy: A practical guide. Ther Adv Neurol Disord. 2022;15:17562864221101687.
27. Bruno E, Maira G, Biondi A, Richardson MP; RADAR-CNS Consortium. Ictal hypoxemia: A systematic review and meta-analysis. Seizure. 2018;63:7-13.
28. Pennell PB, Karanam A, Meador KJ, Gerard E, Kalayjian L, Penovich P, et al. Antiseizure medication concentrations during pregnancy: Results from the Maternal Outcomes and Neurodevelopmental Effects of Antiepileptic Drugs (MONEAD) Study. JAMA Neurol. 2022;79(4):370-9.
29. McElrath TF, Druzin M, Van Marter LJ, May RC, Brown C, Stek A, et al. The obstetrical care and delivery experience of women with epilepsy in the MONEAD Study. Am J Perinatol. 2024;41(7):935-43.
30. Pack AM, Oskoui M, Williams Roberson S, Donley DK, French J, Gerard EE, et al. Teratogenesis, perinatal, and neurodevelopmental outcomes after in utero exposure to antiseizure medication: Practice guideline from the AAN, AES, and SMFM. Neurology. 2024;102(11):e209279.
31. Parker SE, Yazdy MM, Mitchell AA, Demmer LA, Werler MM. A description of spina bifida cases and co-occurring malformations, 1976-2011. Am J Med Genet A. 2014;164A(2):432-40.
32. Smithells RW, Sheppard S, Schorah CJ, Seller MJ, Nevin NC, Harris R, et al. Apparent prevention of neural tube defects by periconceptional vitamin supplementation. Arch Dis Child. 1981;56(12):911-8.
33. Ban L, Fleming KM, Doyle P, Smeeth L, Hubbard RB, Fiaschi L, et al. Congenital anomalies in children of mothers taking antiepileptic drugs with and without periconceptional high dose folic acid use: A population-based cohort study. PLoS One. 2015;10(7):e0131130.
34. Tomson T, Battino D, Bonizzoni E, Craig J, Lindhout D, Perucca E, et al.; EURAP Study Group. Comparative risk of major congenital malformations with eight different antiepileptic drugs: A prospective cohort study of the EURAP registry. Lancet Neurol. 2018;17(6):530-8.
35. Baker GA, Bromley RL, Briggs M, Cheyne CP, Cohen MJ, García-Fiñana M, et al. IQ at 6 years after in utero exposure to antiepileptic drugs: A controlled cohort study. Neurology. 2015;84(4):382-90.
36. Kasradze S, Gogatishvili N, Lomidze G, Ediberidze T, Lazariashvili M, Khomeriki K, et al. Cognitive functions in children exposed to antiepileptic drugs in utero: Study in Georgia. Epilepsy Behav. 2017;66:105-12.
37. Bjørk M, Riedel B, Spigset O, Veiby G, Kolstad E, Daltveit AK, et al. Association of folic acid supplementation during pregnancy with the risk of autistic traits in children exposed to antiepileptic drugs in utero. JAMA Neurol. 2018;75(2):160-8.
38. Husebye ESN, Gilhus NE, Riedel B, Spigset O, Daltveit AK, Bjørk MH. Verbal abilities in children of mothers with epilepsy: Association to maternal folate status. Neurology. 2018;91(9):e811-21.
39. Meador KJ, Baker GA, Browning N, Clayton-Smith J, Combs-Cantrell DT, Cohen M, et al. Cognitive function at 3 years of age after fetal exposure to antiepileptic drugs. N Engl J Med. 2009;360(16):1597-605.
40. Bjørk MH, Tomson T, Dreier JW, Alvestad S, Gilhus NE, Gissler M, et al. High-dose folic acid and cancer risk; unjustified concerns by von Wrede

and colleagues regarding our paper. Epilepsia. 2023;64(9):2244-8.
41. Birnbaum AK, Meador KJ, Karanam A, Brown C, May RC, Gerard EE, et al. Antiepileptic drug exposure in infants of breastfeeding mothers with epilepsy. JAMA Neurol. 2020;77(4):441-50.
42. Shawahna R, Zaid L. Concentrations of antiseizure medications in breast milk of lactating women with epilepsy: A systematic review with qualitative synthesis. Seizure. 2022;98:57-70.
43. Drugs and Lactation Database (LactMed®). [Internet]. Bethesda (MD): National Institute of Child Health and Human Development; 2006.
44. Kim H, Faught E, Thurman DJ, Fishman J, Kalilani L. Antiepileptic drug treatment patterns in women of childbearing age with epilepsy. JAMA Neurol. 2019;76(7):783-90.
45. Meador KJ, Baker GA, Browning N, Cohen MJ, Bromley RL, Clayton-Smith J, et al. Fetal antiepileptic drug exposure and cognitive outcomes at age 6 years (NEAD study): A prospective observational study. Lancet Neurol. 2013;12(3):244-52.
46. Betchel NT, Fariba KA, Saadabadi A. Lamotrigine. In: StatPearls [Internet]. Treasure Island (FL): StatPearls Publishing; 2024 Available from http://www.ncbi.nlm.nih.gov/books/NBK470442/ [Last accessed September, 2024].
47. Johannessen SI, Helde G, Brodtkorb E. Levetiracetam Concentrations in Serum and in Breast Milk at Birth and during Lactation. Epilepsia. 2005;46(5):775-7.
48. Veiby G, Bjørk M, Engelsen BA, Gilhus NE. Epilepsy and recommendations for breastfeeding. Seizure. 2015;28:57-65.
49. Honybun E, Cockle E, Malpas CB, O'Brien TJ, Vajda FJ, Perucca P, et al. Neurodevelopmental and functional outcomes following in utero exposure to antiseizure medication: A Systematic Review. Neurology. 202;102(8):e209175.
50. Jentink J, Loane MA, Dolk H, Barisic I, Garne E, Morris JK, et al. Valproic acid monotherapy in pregnancy and major congenital malformations. N Engl J Med. 2010;362(23):2185-93.
51. Christensen J, Grønborg TK, Sørensen MJ, Schendel D, Parner ET, Pedersen LH, et al. Prenatal valproate exposure and risk of autism spectrum disorders and childhood autism. JAMA. 2013;309(16):1696-703.
52. Coste J, Blotiere PO, Miranda S, Mikaeloff Y, Peyre H, Ramus F, et al. Risk of early neurodevelopmental disorders associated with in utero exposure to valproate and other antiepileptic drugs: A nationwide cohort study in France. Sci Rep. 2020;10(1):17362.
53. Dreier JW, Bjørk MH, Alvestad S, Gissler M, Igland J, Leinonen MK, et al. Prenatal exposure to antiseizure medication and incidence of childhood- and adolescence-onset psychiatric disorders. JAMA Neurol. 2023;80(6):568-77.
54. Pal DK, Pong AW, Chung WK. Genetic evaluation and counseling for epilepsy. Nat Rev Neurol. 2010;6(8):445-53.
55. Camfield CS, Striano P, Camfield PR. Epidemiology of juvenile myoclonic epilepsy. Epilepsy Behav. 2013;28(Suppl 1):S15-7.
56. Marson AG, Al-Kharusi AM, Alwaidh M, Appleton R, Baker GA, Chadwick DW, et al. The SANAD study of effectiveness of valproate, lamotrigine, or topiramate for generalised and unclassifiable epilepsy: An unblinded randomised controlled trial. Lancet. 2007;369(9566):1016-26.
57. Marson A, Burnside G, Appleton R, Smith D, Leach JP, Sills G, et al. The SANAD II study of the effectiveness and cost-effectiveness of valproate versus levetiracetam for newly diagnosed generalised and unclassifiable epilepsy: An open-label, non-inferiority, multicentre, phase 4, randomised controlled trial. Lancet. 2021;397(10282):1375-86.
58. Cerulli Irelli E, Cocchi E, Morano A, Gesche J, Caraballo RH, Lattanzi S, et al. Predictors of seizure recurrence in women with idiopathic generalized epilepsy who switch from valproate to another medication. Neurology. 2024;102(9):e209222.
59. Farmen AH, Grundt JH, Tomson T, Nakken KO, Nakling J, Mowinchel P, et al. Age-specific birth rates in women with epilepsy: A population-based study. Brain Behav. 2016;6(8):e00492.
60. Pennell PB, French JA, Harden CL, Davis A, Bagiella E, Andreopoulos E, et al. Fertility and birth outcomes in women with epilepsy seeking pregnancy. JAMA Neurol. 2018;75(8):962-9.
61. Sukumaran SC, Sarma PS, Thomas SV. Polytherapy increases the risk of infertility in women with epilepsy. Neurology. 2010;75(15):1351-5.
62. Larsen MD, Jølving LR, Fedder J, Nørgård BM. The efficacy of assisted reproductive treatment in women with epilepsy. Reprod Biomed Online. 2020;41(6):1015-22.
63. Gerard EE, Haut S, Patel P, Sazgar M. Change in seizure pattern and menopause. In: Sazgar M, Harden CL (Eds). Controversies in Caring for Women with Epilepsy: Sorting Through the Evidence [Internet]. Cham: Springer International Publishing; 2016. pp. 141-52. Available from:

https://doi.org/10.1007/978-3-319-29170-3_17 [Last accessed September, 2024].
64. Guo Y, Lin Z, Huang Y, Yu L. Effects of valproate, lamotrigine, and levetiracetam monotherapy on bone health in newly diagnosed adult patients with epilepsy. Epilepsy Behav. 2020;113:107489.
65. Carvalho V, Colonna I, Curia G, Ferretti MT, Arabia G, Molnar MJ, et al. Sex steroid hormones and epilepsy: Effects of hormonal replacement therapy on seizure frequency of postmenopausal women with epilepsy—A systematic review. Eur J Neurol. 2023;30(9):2884-98.
66. Harden CL, Herzog AG, Nikolov BG, Koppel BS, Christos PJ, Fowler K, et al. Hormone replacement therapy in women with epilepsy: A randomized, double-blind, placebo-controlled study. Epilepsia. 2006;47(9):1447-51.
67. National Institute for Health and care Excellence. (2012). Osteoporosis: Assessing the risk of fragility fracture. Clinical guideline. [online]. Available from https://www.nice.org.uk/guidance/cg146 [Last accessed September, 2024.]
68. Awasthi H, Mani D, Singh D, Gupta A. The underlying pathophysiology and therapeutic approaches for osteoporosis. Med Res Rev. 2018;38(6):2024-57.
69. Kinariwalla N, Sen A. The psychosocial impact of epilepsy on marriage: A narrative review. Epilepsy Behav. 2016;63:34-41.
70. Tellez-Zenteno JF, Patten SB, Jetté N, Williams J, Wiebe S. Psychiatric comorbidity in epilepsy: A population-based analysis. Epilepsia. 2007;48(12):2336-44.
71. Goldstein LH, Robinson EJ, Reuber M, Chalder T, Callaghan H, Eastwood C, et al. Characteristics of 698 patients with dissociative seizures: A UK multicenter study. Epilepsia. 2019;60(11):2182-93.
72. Karan V, Harsha S, Keshava BS, Pradeep R, Sathyanarayana Rao TS, Andrade C. Sexual dysfunction in women with epilepsy. Indian J Psychiatry. 2015;57(3):301-4.
73. Kalmbach DA, Pillai V, Kingsberg SA, Ciesla JA. The transaction between depression and anxiety symptoms and sexual functioning: A prospective study of premenopausal, healthy women. Arch Sex Behav. 2015;44(6):1635-49.
74. Josephson CB, Jetté N. Psychiatric comorbidities in epilepsy. Int Rev Psychiatry. 2017;29(5):409-24.
75. Verboket RD, Söhling N, Marzi I, Paule E, Knake S, Rosenow F, et al. Prevalence, risk factors and therapeutic aspects of injuries and accidents in women with epilepsy. Eur J Trauma Emerg Surg. 2019;45(3):375-81.
76. Kanner AM, Ribot R, Mazarati A. Bidirectional relations among common psychiatric and neurologic comorbidities and epilepsy: Do they have an impact on the course of the seizure disorder? Epilepsia Open. 2018;3:210-9.
77. Spina E, Pisani F, de Leon J. Clinically significant pharmacokinetic drug interactions of antiepileptic drugs with new antidepressants and new antipsychotics. Pharmacol Res. 2016;106: 72-86.
78. Mula M. The pharmacological management of psychiatric comorbidities in patients with epilepsy. Pharmacol Res. 2016;107:147-53.
79. Wu CS, Wang SC, Yeh IJ, Liu SK. Comparative risk of seizure with use of first- and second-generation antipsychotics in patients with schizophrenia and mood disorders. J Clin Psychiatry. 2016;77(5): e573-9.

CHAPTER 4

The Art and Science of Choosing and Combining Antiseizure Medications

Parampreet Singh Kharbanda

ABSTRACT

All types of seizures do not respond equally to all antiseizure medications (ASMs), and these ASMs have many different side effects. Some types of seizures can even worsen with specific ASMs. Hence, the correct choice of ASMs and their combinations are important parts of drug therapy for the control of seizures. Knowing how to do this properly has become even more significant due to the high number of new medications added to the group in the last few years. Although a complete and comprehensive review of all the ASMs is not in the purview of this chapter, the common clinically relevant factors affecting the choice of the appropriate ASMs are discussed. These factors deciding the choice of ASMs include the type of seizures, type of epilepsy, side effects, drug interactions, comorbidities, cost, and more are detailed in the chapter. Treatment with a single ASM gives the best outcome, but in a group of patients, this is not enough to control the seizures effectively. Hence, the ASM needs to be changed, or a new ASM is added to the ongoing regimen. There are many considerations for combining two or more ASMs; these are mainly the seizure type, side effects of ASMs, mechanism of action, and drug interactions. Finally, if the seizure type remains unclassified initially in a given patient, either due to vague semiology or nonavailability of witnessed history, a suitable broad-spectrum efficacy ASM can be started until further information is available.

Keywords: Antiseizure medications, Choosing antiseizure medications, Antiseizure medication combinations.

■ INTRODUCTION

Epilepsy is a unique disorder, unlike any other. This is probably the only illness where a person may have just one myoclonic jerk and an abnormal electroencephalogram (EEG) and may end up taking lifelong treatment, even though you may never have any other symptom in your life.

Once we have established that it was an epileptic seizure, the choice of antiseizure medications (ASMs) can be both simple and complex. It can be simple, at least, for the initial seizure management, even if we cannot classify the seizures accurately, if we know which ASMs to use in such a scenario. It becomes more complex when the response to the first ASM is suboptimal. A consultation from a comprehensive epilepsy care program may be advisable for such patients. This chapter will focus on some of the practical aspects of choosing the appropriate ASM, whether in monotherapy or in combination, in adults with epilepsy. It will combine facts from published literature with personal experience and opinion. The reader is advised to refer to appropriate publications, including the ones referenced in this chapter, and prescribing information for a comprehensive understanding of the structure, pharmacokinetics, efficacy, and adverse effects of all the ASMs.

■ ROLE OF ANTISEIZURE MEDICATIONS

The end goal for drug treatment of epilepsy is to improve or sustain the quality of life of the patients. This is achieved mainly through effective control of seizures while minimizing the incidence of adverse effects. The role of ASMs in epilepsy management is largely limited to control of seizures, meaning that it is symptomatic therapy. We are still awaiting effective antiepileptogenic medications, which can help prevent the development of epilepsy after the causative insult to the brain, by having some kind of disease-modifying effect.

The biggest limitation of ASMs is their failure to control all the seizures in a significant percentage of patients, many of which end up having drug-resistant epilepsy (DRE). It is noteworthy that most of the ASMs fail in the same group of patients. Though a small percentage of DRE patients respond to previously untried combinations, most do not respond to any ASM. This makes us think that the resistance to ASMs is not about the drug, it is likely to be a characteristic of the epilepsy itself.

■ COMMON ANTISEIZURE MEDICATIONS

A complete review of all the ASMs is not in the purview of this chapter. We will have a brief description of common ASMs, mainly focusing on their place in our current algorithm for drug treatment of epilepsy. This includes some salient features including indications, contraindications, drug interactions, and some of the common adverse effects, relevant to making a choice of the appropriate ASM. An ideal ASM would be the one which controls all the seizures in the given patient without having adverse effects or undesired drug interactions.

Levetiracetam

Levetiracetam has become the go-to drug in many types of seizures and various situations due to its unique properties. This is mainly because of its near-inert character combined with a broad spectrum of efficacy in nearly all types of seizures. It does not induce hepatic enzymes, and more importantly, does not get affected significantly when combined with enzyme-inducing ASMs. Hence, it is a great drug for combination therapy. Levetiracetam can be started immediately at the starting level maintenance dose and has a parenteral formulation where needed, making it useful in both acute and chronic epilepsy treatment. To add to that, it is one of the safest ASMs in pregnancy.[1] Hence, levetiracetam ticks most of the boxes for being an ideal ASM. However, it is not perfect. A significant minority, roughly around 15%, of patients experience psychiatric side effects, especially the ones with preexisting intellectual disabilities.[2] This makes it difficult to use in such patients, and those who already have a psychiatric comorbidity. It remains the drug of choice in women with generalized epilepsies, particularly those with child-bearing potential. It is one of the main ASMs for the treatment of status epilepticus. Levetiracetam binds to synaptic vesicle protein SV2A, though the exact mechanism of action (MOA) is unclear.

Carbamazepine

Carbamazepine holds the title of being one of the most effective, if not "the" most effective

ASM for focal seizures, especially focal with impaired awareness seizures. It is one of the cheapest ASMs, at least in our setup. It needs to be started slowly due to the phenomenon of autoinduction, thus it takes some time to achieve a steady state of metabolism. It induces the cytochrome P450 (CYP) system hepatic enzymes and can increase the metabolism of other drugs, including ASMs which are metabolized by this pathway. It belongs to the group of ASMs which can cause skin rash of mild-to-serious nature (toxic epidermal necrolysis and Stevens–Johnson syndrome).[3] Hence, screening for HLA-B*1502 allele is recommended in Asian ancestry patients. All patients being started on carbamazepine should be counseled regarding the risk of the rash; otherwise, many patients may not know why they have developed the rash, and not seek immediate redressal including discontinuation of the offending drug. Carbamazepine works by binding to voltage-dependent sodium channels.

Valproate

Valproate (valproic acid) is the true broad-spectrum drug with efficacy in almost all known types of seizures. It is probably the most effective drug for primary generalized tonic–clonic seizures, myoclonic seizures, absence seizures (along with ethosuximide), and has good efficacy in focal seizures too. It does not induce hepatic enzymes; in fact, it moderately inhibits the CYP system to an extent. Valproate may have a mood-stabilizing effect, which may be beneficial in patients with psychiatric comorbidity. However, there are multiple issues in using this ASM in women with epilepsy, including but not limited to, one of the highest incidences of major malformations in the offspring exposed to this drug in utero. You can find more details on this topic in the chapter "Management of Women with Epilepsy" in this book. The common side effects include weight gain, tremor, and loss of hair. It can give rise to hyperammonemic encephalopathy, which can be serious in some cases, so this needs to be considered in patients on valproate who present with unexplained encephalopathy.[4] Still, it remains the drug of choice in most men with primary generalized epilepsies. Its antiseizure effects are mediated through multiple mechanisms.

Clobazam

Clobazam is a benzodiazepine used as an add-on in the management of DRE. It has a fast onset of action. Hence, it is a useful drug for intermittent use for periods with escalation of seizure frequency, or as a bridging drug when ASMs are being switched. It is also used in catamenial seizures.[5] Its MOA is binding to the gamma-aminobutyric acid type A (GABA-A) receptor.

Oxcarbazepine

Oxcarbazepine is related to carbamazepine in its structure, spectrum, and efficacy, with some notable differences. It is not a strong hepatic enzyme inducer, and thus a better drug for combination therapy. It does not have autoinduction and can be started at doses of 300–600 mg/day. It is a slightly better tolerated alternative to carbamazepine if affordability is not an issue. However, it has a higher incidence of hyponatremia than carbamazepine. The risk of serious skin reactions is lesser than carbamazepine.[6] HLA-B*1502 allele testing has been suggested in Asian ethnicity populations.

Lamotrigine

Lamotrigine is one of the best-tolerated ASMs, with its low incidence of neurocognitive effects. It is a reasonably broad-spectrum ASM, with good efficacy in focal and also some generalized seizures, especially absence seizures. It has been known to precipitate myoclonus in some patients with juvenile myoclonic epilepsy. It works well in combination therapy, except with some hormonal contraceptives.[7] It is one of the safest ASMs in pregnancy, but the serum levels may fall significantly in the later period of gestation. It has a tendency to cause skin rash, and patients need to be advised to look for skin rash and manage it as mentioned under carbamazepine earlier. It is not a good drug for acute control of seizures as it needs many weeks to be introduced in therapeutic doses. The MOA of lamotrigine is not fully known but possibly includes inactivating voltage-dependent sodium channels.

Topiramate

Topiramate is a good drug to use when migraine is comorbid with epilepsy, due to its efficacy in both. It is an ASM that usually is used as a second-line drug in the management of generalized epilepsies as it has a broad spectrum of efficacy. We try to keep the maximum dose under 400 mg/day, as higher doses can have side effects like impaired expressive language and cognition.[8] It is associated with kidney stones in a small percentage of patients, so the history of the same needs to be elicited in the patient and their family before prescribing topiramate. A welcome effect in many patients is the lack of weight gain and even some weight loss while using topiramate.[9] It acts through multiple mechanisms.

Lacosamide

Lacosamide is used in the management of focal seizures, both as monotherapy and as an add-on. It is a well-tolerated drug and does not significantly induce hepatic enzymes. It may be a good option where a sodium channel ASM is required to be used in combination therapy. It works mainly by slow inactivation of voltage-dependent sodium channels.

Perampanel

Perampanel is one of the recent additions to the ASM armamentarium. In our setup, it comes in handy as an add-on in DRE. It can be used as a once-a-day dose. It has a tendency to cause psychiatric adverse effects at the higher end of dose spectrum. It has a unique MOA as an alpha-amino-3-hydroxy-5-methyl-4-isoxazolepropionic acid (AMPA)-type glutamate receptor antagonist.

Brivaracetam

Brivaracetam is very similar in mechanism, spectrum, and efficacy to levetiracetam. However, it has a different pharmacokinetics and is partly metabolized in liver through CYP2C19 enzyme, thereby making it more amenable to drug interactions than levetiracetam.[10] There is some evidence that it may have lesser psychiatric effects than levetiracetam. In our setup, levetiracetam still remains the initial choice out of the two, due to the long experience with this drug, especially in patients who do not have risk factors for higher psychiatric side effects.

Ethosuximide

Ethosuximide is a narrow-spectrum ASM, mainly limited to its effect on absence seizures. It has similar efficacy to valproate in controlling absences but is better tolerated than valproate. It acts by diminishing the T-type calcium currents in thalamic neurons.

Eslicarbazepine

Eslicarbazepine is an active metabolite of oxcarbazepine (S-licarbazepine) and also has similar spectrum of efficacy to its prodrug. It has the benefit of once-a-day dosing.

Phenytoin and Fosphenytoin

Phenytoin, another sodium channel blocker, was the mainstay for the management of focal seizures in the past. It has nonlinear kinetics, and hence its clearance and half-life fluctuate with plasma concentration. Because of this, and some common side effects like gum hyperplasia, currently, we use it mainly as a backup drug for focal seizures. It can be administrated through parenteral route (preferably as its prodrug fosphenytoin), and hence can be used for acute control of seizures. It is a potent inducer of the CYP system.

Zonisamide

We use zonisamide mainly as an add-on for resistant primary generalized seizures, due to its efficacy in controlling myoclonic seizures. However, it is a broad-spectrum ASM and can be used for focal seizures too. The main MOA seems to be by blocking T-type calcium channels, along with voltage-dependent sodium channels.

■ FACTORS AFFECTING ANTISEIZURE MEDICATION CHOICE

There has been a spurt in the number of new ASMs in the last two decades. Where it has helped us have more options at our disposal to choose from, none of them has yet shown the potential of controlling seizures in all the patients, or being totally devoid of unwanted effects. This has also made it imperative for practitioners to have good working knowledge of the indications, contraindications, and other special features of these ASMs, so that they can make the best therapeutic choice for a given situation. There are multiple factors that influence this choice, some of which are listed here and dealt with in detail following that:
- Type of seizures
- Type of epilepsy
- Side effects
- Speed of initiation
- Drug interactions
- Elimination
- Frequency of dosing
- Special situations
- Comorbidities
- Patient preferences
- Cost

Type of Seizures

As expected, the type of seizure is the main determinant of the choice of ASM. This is because some types of seizures respond preferentially to specific ASMs. This is more relevant for primary generalized seizures, especially myoclonic and absence seizures. They respond to only a few of the ASMs and can actually worsen with inappropriately used ASMs **(Table 1)**.

Type of Epilepsy

Type of epilepsy is also a consideration when choosing ASMs. Different epilepsies present with either a single type of seizure or a combination of seizure types. Epilepsies that have more than one seizure types, e.g., juvenile myoclonic epilepsy, need to be treated with ASMs that can control all their inherent seizure types; like in this case, bilateral tonic-clonic and myoclonic seizures. The ability to control a particular type of seizure, e.g., bilateral tonic–clonic, may differ depending upon the type of epilepsy they are associated with. Carbamazepine may effectively control the bilateral tonic-clonic seizures in a temporal lobe epilepsy but may fail to have the same effect on this seizure type when they are part of juvenile myoclonic epilepsy.

Side Effects

Adverse effects are as common a reason for ASM discontinuation as is the failure of efficacy. These effects can be neurotoxic or systemic. An important point to keep

TABLE 1: Preferred and avoidable drugs according to seizure types in our practice.

Seizure type	Preferred antiseizure medications (ASM)	Backup ASMs	Drug-resistant epilepsy (DRE)
Focal aware Focal impaired awareness Focal to bilateral tonic–clonic	• Carbamazepine • Oxcarbazepine • Lamotrigine • Levetiracetam	• Lacosamide • Brivaracetam • Phenytoin • Valproate • Clobazam • Eslicarbazepine • Perampanel • Topiramate	Phenobarbitone
Generalized onset tonic–clonic (GTCS) Myoclonic + GTCS	• Valproate (males) • Levetiracetam (females)	• Brivaracetam • Topiramate	• Clobazam • Zonisamide • Perampanel
Absence	Ethosuximide	• Valproate • Lamotrigine	
Absences + GTCS	Valproate	• Lamotrigine • Levetiracetam	Topiramate
Unclassified	• Levetiracetam • Valproate	• Lamotrigine • Topiramate • Brivaracetam	Clobazam
Seizure type and epilepsies • Myoclonic • Absence • Idiopathic and genetic generalized epilepsies	ASMs to avoid • Carbamazepine • Oxcarbazepine • Phenytoin • Vigabatrin • Gabapentin		

in mind is that clinical toxicity can occur even when the serum levels of the ASM are normal. Adverse effects are never welcome, but if one is able to initially tolerate them for a few weeks, many of these will wane off over time. Almost all ASMs have side effects that can limit their use. However, there may be situations or comorbidities where a particular side effect may need to be avoided. Some professionals who need active cognitive functions may prefer ASMs with minimal sedation, like lamotrigine.

Consider spreading the daily dose over 3–4 times per day to reduce the adverse effects, before abandoning a drug for that reason **(Table 2)**.

Speed of Initiation

Drugs like lamotrigine that are introduced over a few weeks are not suitable for situations where the seizures are very frequent or generalized, or they need to be urgently controlled. If introduced too fast, it can have unwanted side effects, including a higher risk of serious skin rash. Carbamazepine also requires a couple of weeks to reach the full maintenance dose.

TABLE 2: Some common and unique side effects of antiseizure medications (ASMs).

Unique side effects	ASMs most commonly associated
Psychiatric and behavioral	• Perampanel • Levetiracetam • Brivaracetam
Bone marrow suppression	Carbamazepine
Hair loss	Valproate
• Weight loss • Kidney stones • Expressive language dysfunction	Topiramate
Sexual dysfunction in males	• Carbamazepine • Phenytoin
Hyponatremia	• Oxcarbazepine • Eslicarbazepine • Carbamazepine
Gingival hypertrophy	Phenytoin
Positive effects	
Efficacy in migraine	Topiramate
Efficacy in mood stabilization	Valproate

Drug Interactions

When the patient is already on other medications for various illnesses, the potential interactions of ASMs with those drugs should be considered. It is imperative that we know if the levels of ASM are going to be increased or lowered by the comedication, and vice versa, so that dose corrections can be made, to avoid failure of efficacy or enhanced adverse effects. These situations may also be an indication of ASM-level monitoring.

Elimination

Route of elimination is another factor deciding the choice of ASM. For example, ASMs like levetiracetam, with predominantly renal elimination, would need to have their doses modified in patients with significant renal impairment. Similarly, drugs like valproate may be avoided in liver damage, and other ASMs which are metabolized in liver may need to be closely monitored.

Frequency of Dosing

Depending on their half-lives, ASMs can be taken once, twice, or thrice a day. This frequency of dosing can have a bearing on the choice of ASM. Patient compliance may be better with lesser number of doses in a day. This is especially true for ASMs that need to be given thrice a day, as the mid-day dose may be the one which may be missed most frequently due to the patient being at work or school, or forgetting to carry it along.[11] Hence, extended-release preparations of such drugs are preferred, which can be taken twice a day.

Special Situations

There are many special situations where the ASM regimen may need to be tweaked. These include management of epilepsy in the elderly population and in pregnant women. The management in old people is discussed in detail in the chapter "Epilepsy Management in the Elderly" in this book. Other situations like hepatic and renal impairment have been dealt with in different sections of this chapter.

Comorbidities

There may be certain comorbidities where a particular ASM may be beneficial, or problematic. For example, patients with comorbid migraine may benefit from using topiramate. Similarly, valproate may be a good drug if the patient also has mood disorders, but it may not be a choice for seizures in the setting of mitochondrial disorders. Drugs like valproate, carbamazepine, lamotrigine, etc., may not be best for patients with diagnosed cardiac rhythm disorders. Topiramate may not be prescribed in patients with a history of renal stones.

Patient Preferences

Sometimes, patients may prefer to take or avoid specific ASMs based on their side effects, cost, or other lifestyle factors. We have seen this among women contemplating pregnancy. They may have their own thoughts on how to balance the risk of seizure with the adverse effects on the fetus. Other situations where patients may like to exercise their choice may be related to the cognitive effects of the medication versus the seizure control. These situations will need thorough discussion with patients to help them make a well-informed decision of their choice. People with a very active lifestyle may want to tailor their ASM regimen so as to have adequate cover for expected intermittent seizure-provoking factors like sleep deprivation.

Cost of Therapy

The cost of therapy is important in settings where patients pay out of their pocket for the ASMs. Their monthly income should be factored in while choosing the right ASM, so that there is less chance of drug default due to inability to afford specific ASMs.

Something that needs to be kept in mind is that though the above recommendations are mostly based on research evidence, in practice it is not rare to find patients who are well-controlled on ASMs that may not be ideal for the said diagnosis. Whether they denote some outliers or overlapping syndromes may not be fully clear. Sometimes we may need to look at the EEG to rule out subclinical epileptiform activity, leading to a decision to change the ASM to a more appropriate one.

■ COMBINATION THERAPY

About half of the drug-naïve epilepsy patients achieve seizure freedom with the first appropriately chosen ASM use. After the failure of the first ASM, the chance to render the patient seizure-free significantly decreases with every additional add-on medication **(Fig. 1)**.[12] However, combinations are beneficial in many patients with DRE, especially the ones who are not candidates for epilepsy surgery. Usually, the decision to add another ASM is made when the first ASM is effective, but not able to render the patient completely seizure-free at the tolerated dose. The factors taken into consideration while choosing the ASM to add-on to the ongoing regimen mainly include efficacy, side effects, and drug interactions.

Factors Affecting Antiseizure Medication Combination

Some of the factors are the same as when choosing the first ASM. However, there are some other determinants that need to be considered when an add-on antiseizure drug is to be added to the current regimen. These are discussed below.

Efficacy in Specific Seizure Types

Even while combining two ASMs, the most important determinant of the choice of ASM remains their efficacy in the specific seizure types and epilepsy of the given patient.

Mechanism of Action

It is preferable to combine ASMs with different MOA; as combining ASMs with similar MOA may sometimes lead to additive adverse effects, without conferring much benefit in efficacy. Combining ASMs with different MOA can provide a better and broader coverage. This is especially beneficial in people who have multiple types of seizures or unclassified seizures.

Side Effects

A patient with a history of skin rash with a past antiseizure drug should avoid using another ASMs that commonly cause skin rash, as there is significant cross-reactivity between these agents. Two drugs that cause

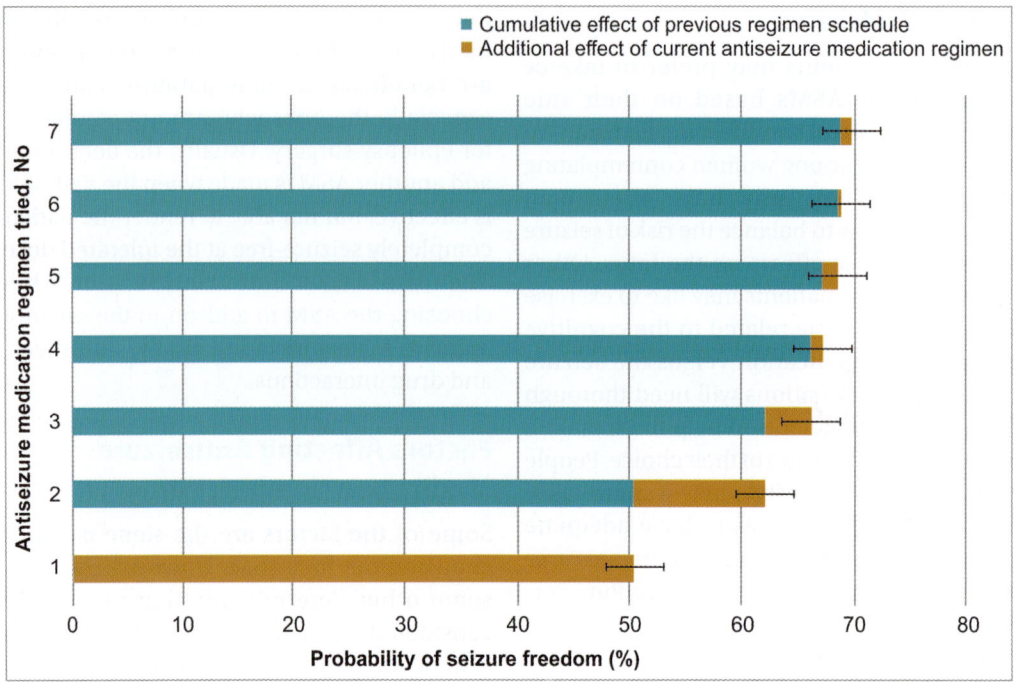

FIG. 1: Seizure freedom with every additional antiseizure medication (ASM) regimen.

psychiatric side effects (e.g., levetiracetam and perampanel) should ideally not be combined.

Drug Interactions

Drug–drug interactions are one of the most important considerations when combining two ASMs. A lot depends upon how the combined ASMs act. They could either be additive, supra-additive, or infra-additive in efficacy and cause enhanced adverse effects when combined. They could increase or drastically decrease the serum levels of the other ASM in the combination. Hepatic enzyme-inducing ASMs if used in combination will decrease the levels of other drugs which are metabolized in liver. For example, Valproate increases the lamotrigine levels when they are used in combination, leading to lesser doses of lamotrigine required to get the same serum levels **(Box 1)**.

BOX 1: Ideal and nonideal combinations of antiseizure medications (ASMs).

- *Group 1:* Hepatic enzyme inducers
- *Group 2:* Non/weak inducers of hepatic enzymes
- *Group 3:* Amenable to induction (hepatic metabolized)
- *Group 4:* Not/minimally amenable to induction (not significantly hepatic metabolized)

ASM combinations in order of preference: Groups 4+4 or 2+4 > 2+3 > 1+3.

Avoid if possible: 1+1

■ CONCLUSION

The art and science of choosing ASMs can be complex. However, if we are aware of the unique properties of the various ASMs and their indications, we can get it right in most patients.

REFERENCES

1. Tomson T, Battino D, Bonizzoni E, Craig J, Lindhout D, Perucca E, et al. Comparative risk of major congenital malformations with eight different antiepileptic drugs: A prospective cohort study of the EURAP registry. Lancet Neurol. 2018;17(6): 530-8.
2. Hurtado B, Koepp MJ, Sander JW, Thompson PJ. The impact of levetiracetam on challenging behavior. Epilepsy Behav. 2006;8(3):588-92.
3. Arif H, Buchsbaum R, Weintraub D, Koyfman S, Salas-Humara C, Bazil CW, et al. Comparison and predictors of rash associated with 15 antiepileptic drugs. Neurology. 2007;68(20):1701-9.
4. Wu J, Li J, Jing W, Tian X, Wang X. Valproic acid-induced encephalopathy: A review of clinical features, risk factors, diagnosis, and treatment. Epilepsy Behav. 2021;120:107967.
5. Maguire MJ, Nevitt SJ. Treatments for seizures in catamenial (menstrual-related) epilepsy. Cochrane Database Syst Rev. 2021;2021(9):CD013225.
6. Chen CB, Hsiao YH, Wu T, Hsih MS, Tassaneeyakul W, Jorns TP, et al. Risk and association of HLA with oxcarbazepine-induced cutaneous adverse reactions in Asians. Neurology. 2017;88(1):78-86.
7. Contin M, Albani F, Ambrosetto G, Avoni P, Bisulli F, Riva R, et al. Variation in lamotrigine plasma concentrations with hormonal contraceptive monthly cycles in patients with epilepsy. Epilepsia. 2006;47(9):1573-5.
8. Cirulli ET, Urban TJ, Marino SE, Linney KN, Birnbaum AK, Depondt C, et al. Genetic and environmental correlates of topiramate-induced cognitive impairment. Epilepsia. 2012;53(1): e5-8.
9. Ben-Menachem E, Axelsen M, Johanson EH, Stagge A, Smith U. Predictors of weight loss in adults with topiramate-treated epilepsy. Obes Res. 2003;11(4):556-62.
10. Hagemann A, Klimpel D, Bien CG, Brandt C, May TW. Influence of dose and antiepileptic comedication on brivaracetam serum concentrations in patients with epilepsy. Epilepsia. 2020;61(5):e43.
11. Singh P, Gupta K, Singh G, Kaushal S. A prospective observational study to assess compliance and factors influencing compliance with antiepileptic drugs among patients with epilepsy. IJBCP. 2019;8(8):1838-43.
12. Chen Z, Brodie MJ, Liew D, Kwan P. Treatment outcomes in patients with newly diagnosed epilepsy treated with established and new antiepileptic drugs: A 30-year longitudinal cohort study. JAMA Neurol. 2018;75(3):279-86.

CHAPTER 5

Medical Management of Drug-resistant Epilepsy

Bharat Kumar Sahu, Swapan Gupta

> **ABSTRACT**
>
> Management of drug-resistant epilepsy is primarily surgical but when surgical option is either contraindicated or failed, continuing medical management is the only option available. Holistic approach for the medical management of drug-resistant epilepsy is crucial. Wrong diagnosis, drug, and dosing are important reasons for pseudoresistance and must be ruled out. Preventable seizure triggers like irregular food, sleep, stress, and fever should be adequately addressed. Compliance must be ensured by more frequent physician visits, medication chart or pill count, longer drug dose intervals, and use of extended-release preparations. Combination drugs can be tried from different classes with different mechanisms of action. This is rational polytherapy. Novel therapeutics including precision medicine, targeted drug delivery, and pharmacogenomic-guided therapy can further help circumvent drug resistance in such patients. Additionally, dietary changes and addressing comorbid conditions also play important role in management of these patients.
>
> **Keywords:** Drug-resistant epilepsy, Refractory epilepsy, Anti-epileptic drug therapy, Medical management, Rational polytherapy.

■ INTRODUCTION

Drug-resistant epilepsy (DRE) is defined as failure of two or more appropriately chosen antiseizure medications (ASMs) either singly or in combination in appropriate dose for a sufficient period of time.[1]

Almost 30% of patients with epilepsy are drug resistant,[2] and out of them almost half are amenable to surgical management. There will also be cases where previous surgical management was tried but either failed or responded poorly. In such cases, the treating physician is rather compelled to continue the medical management of epilepsy. Often such cases are neglected and further options in management strategy are not explored as they are labeled refractory. Patients with DRE and uncontrolled seizures may experience increases in seizure frequency and severity, along with cognitive and psychiatric dysfunction, injuries, status epilepticus, and sudden unexpected death in epilepsy (SUDEP).[3] This chapter will look at the best management approach as per evidence to manage such patients to achieve the best possible outcome. The best possible outcome here would not necessarily mean complete seizure freedom but even reduction in seizure burden and management of comorbid conditions with the aim to improve overall quality of life (QOL) of such patients.

Medical management of drug-resistant epilepsy shall include:
- ASM treatment
- Controlling factors that increase the likelihood of seizure occurrence
- Nonpharmacological treatment
- Management of comorbid conditions

ANTISEIZURE MEDICATION MANAGEMENT

Exclude Drug Pseudoresistance

Even though the definition of DRE excludes drug-related causes of pseudoresistance, every effort should be made to rule them out. It is not uncommon to see that patients are referred to higher centers for presurgical evaluations for DRE but have pseudoresistance.[4] The doctor must rule out wrong diagnosis like nonepileptic events, wrong drug for the type of seizure (e.g., sodium channel blockers for myoclonic epilepsies), and wrong dosage (e.g., underdosing or with use of concomitant enzyme inducers), which may result in pseudo-drug refractoriness.

Principles of Rational Antiseizure Medications Management

In a hospital-based observational study, the first drug therapy was successful in 49.5% of patients and the second drug was successful in 36.7% of the patients. The success rates of drug trials after failure of the first two drugs were significantly lower but were not different among subsequent drug regimens, ranging from 12.5–22.2%.[5] Therefore, the first and second drug trials are likely to be the major determinants of therapeutic outcomes of epilepsy. It might seem that once patient is labeled truly drug-refractory, there is little scope for further change in drug treatment that will yield clinically meaningful benefit. To an extent, this might be true, but with the discovery of newer ASMs with different mechanisms of actions, better tolerability profile, and favorable pharmacodynamic and pharmacokinetic profile including least drug–drug interactions, a significant proportion of "drug-resistant" patients could achieve seizure freedom. In a large multicenter observational study, ASM adjustment was associated with seizure freedom in one of five patients with drug-resistant focal epilepsy.[6] The set of drugs when used together yield most favorable results in terms of seizure freedom and least side effects is known as "rational polytherapy". This concept is not solely based on disease (epilepsy)-oriented therapy but to individual patient-oriented therapy. It means seizure freedom is not always the goal but rather best possible QOL. Although theoretically attractive, the evidence supporting rational polytherapy is sparse and based primarily on animal models and preclinical studies.[7] The clinical studies available are small, provide only imprecise results and low-level evidence, and are usually observational studies or post hoc or subgroup analyses of randomized controlled trials, which can be affected by confounding; these results should be interpreted with caution. Nevertheless, there are few principles of drug treatment in DRE based on evidence which are discussed below:

- If monotherapy fails, combination duo therapy is considered a rational strategy to improve tolerance and treatment persistence rather than shifting to another ASM monotherapy or increasing the dose of preexisting ASM.[8] In a large 20-year longitudinal hospital cohort observational study, seizure freedom with rational polytherapy was additional 8.4%.[2] Another study showed new drug combination therapy had resulted in seizure freedom in additional 28% and >50% seizure reduction in 21% at 1 year.[9]
- The fear of increased side effects with combination is rather more hypothetical

since it is shown that tolerability is more related to drug load than the number of drugs taken.[10] Drug load is the ratio of prescribed daily dose to the defined recommended daily dose.[11] More drug load means more central nervous system (CNS) adverse effects like somnolence, dizziness, imbalance, fatigue, blurred vision, and cognitive impairment. Patients on duo therapy could tolerate higher total drug load >2 than patients on monotherapy <2.[12] Thus, the least effective dose of add-on ASM be initially tried without necessarily achieving therapeutic drug doses or reducing the dose of preexisting ASM if side effects are troublesome with increasing dose of second ASM is recommended.[13] Always the principle of "start low, go slow" should be followed.[14] Although there are hundreds of choices of combination ASMs possible, proper evidence-based guidelines for the most effective and appropriate drug regimens are not available. Few combinations have been found to be better than others. For example, the combination of valproate with lamotrigine is well known to have synergistic effects.[15] It means their combined therapeutic effect is supra-additive than the sum of effect of individual drugs. In rational polytherapy, combination should have supra-additive therapeutic effect while side effects should be infra-additive, i.e., the side effects when combined are less than the sum of the side effects of the two drugs individually.[16]

- It is shown in various studies that combining drugs with different mechanisms of action has better therapeutic index than combination from the group of drugs with similar mechanisms of action.[17] For example, combination of levetiracetam with carbamazepine or levetiracetam with lacosamide has better efficacy than combination of either of phenytoin/carbamazepine/oxcarbazepine/lacosamide.[18] Levetiracetam acts on SV2 receptors while others are sodium channel blockers. Combination of sodium channel blockers are associated with more adverse events and withdrawal than when combined with drug with different mechanism of action.[19] Treatment persistent rates are thus higher with ASM with different mechanism of action and there is decreased risk of therapy discontinuation and lower inpatient admissions and emergency visits.[20] Moreover, the favorable side effect profile and least drug interactions of newer ASMs result in infra-additive side effect profile of the used combination.
- The choice of drug should also be based on comorbidities and patient profile. The least frequency of dosing and drugs with minimal drug interactions are preferred especially in elderly on polytherapy. Those with neuropsychiatric comorbidity should best avoid levetiracetam, topiramate, and zonisamide.
- One important consideration is "how many drugs can be tried as part of rational polypharmacy". It is shown that triple therapy is associated with lower chances of remission. Addition of fourth or fifth ASM is hardly recommended since it results in significant increase in side effects compared to marginal therapeutic benefit.[21,7] One exception to this rule could be more frequent use of three or more ASMs in severe epilepsies like epileptic encephalopathies. For example, in Dravet syndrome, combination of valproate with lamotrigine and clobazam is usually given. This is because controlling seizures is very important because seizures itself lead to neurocognitive regression in such patients. Similarly, in Lennox–Gastaut syndrome (LGS), valproate with lamotrigine (caution with

- predominant myoclonus as lamotrigine can worsen myoclonic seizures) is first tried and then topiramate and clobazam can be used as add on. Other drugs that can be tried are zonisamide, levetiracetam, perampanel, and now recently approved cannabidiol. Polytherapy is rather the rule in epileptic and developmental encephalopathies.
- Seizures manifest through a circadian rhythm, and such knowledge of temporal patterns of seizure occurrence can dictate schedules for ASM individualized to each patient,[22] adjusting drug treatment schedules to achieve higher peak blood levels when seizures are more frequent. To improve night-time breakthrough seizures, the bedtime dose can be increased; to prevent mid-late afternoon breakthrough seizures, an add-on dose can be prescribed in the early afternoon.
- The era of precision medicine targeting the disease pathogenesis directly has revolutionized treatment in cases where epilepsy was usually drug refractory. A good example is Tuberous sclerosis-related epilepsy where cell signaling mammalian target of rapamycin (mTOR) pathway inhibitors like everolimus and rapamycin, which directly affect the disease pathogenesis, result in significant seizure freedom as compared to conventional ASMs. Others include substitution therapies like ketogenic diet (KD) in glucose transporter 1 (GLUT1) and function-based therapies to modify function of ion channels like use of sodium channel blockers in developmental/epileptic encephalopathies due to pathogenic gain of function variants in SCN1A.[23] The cost and availability are limiting factors.
- Newer third-generation ASMs have promising results, though evidence is still growing. Cenobamate is a recently approved third-generation ASM for add-on therapy for focal epilepsy in adults >18 years. It has dual mechanism of action—decreased neuronal excitability by promoting fast and slow inactivation of sodium channels and preferentially inhibit persistent component of sodium channel unit. It also stimulates allosteric modulation of high-affinity gamma-aminobutyric acid type A (GABA-A) receptors at nonbenzodiazepine site.[24] Small series as an add-on in LGS[25] and Dravet syndrome[26] has shown seizure remission rates of 11% and 21% with 200 mg and 400 mg, respectively. Cannabidiol (used as an add-on treatment for LGS, Dravet syndrome, and tuberous sclerosis complex) is an enzyme-inhibiting drug that can increase serum concentrations of the active metabolite of clobazam. This could synergically potentiate the antiseizure efficacy of the combined drugs but may also explain the increased risk of somnolence among patients using these combination therapies. Fenfluramine is another drug that has been tried in Dravet, LGS, and other drug resistant epileptic syndromes.[27] It exerts its action beyond its proserotonergic activity. Another new drug combination tried with good results is valproate and topiramate over valproate monotherapy, especially in absence, atonic and tonic–clonic seizures.[28] Other newer ASMs are eslicarbazepine acetate and zonisamide.
- Finally, pharmacogenomics is emerging as an important consideration while prescribing an ASM. With the availability of almost 30 ASMs as on date, there can be multiple combinations of drugs possible. In the quest to find the best combination, it is practically impossible to try all such combinations in a given patient. Pharmacogenomic testing can tailor this selection and the choice of ASMs can then be individualized with the best combination predicted based on evidence. Though its clinical applicability

Practical Approach to Rational Polytherapy

Here is a quick guide to make a rational selection of ASM in patients with DRE in clinics. If the patient is on a single drug and the drug is at least partially effective and well tolerable, retain the first drug and choose a second drug with either different or multiple mechanism of action considered to show synergistic interactions with the first drug. If the first drug was not effective and poorly tolerable, it may be more appropriate to try a substitution monotherapy. While considering duo therapy, start the second ASM with a low dose and perform slow escalation up till the dose where clinical efficacy is seen. This dose may be lower than the recommended daily dose of the drug. In case seizures recur, the dose can be increased till seizure control or side effects appear. In case the second drug has good efficacy, but side effects become an issue, the dose of first ASM can be reduced to achieve lesser total drug load. If the first duo therapy is not effective, switch to alternative duo therapy choosing another drug with different mechanism of action for the second duo therapy. If the second duo therapy fails or if the first duo therapy was at least partially effective, one may consider triple therapy.

■ CONTROLLING FACTORS THAT INCREASE LIKELIHOOD OF SEIZURE OCCURRENCE

Managing seizure triggers provoking factors: We know drugs are the mainstay to control seizures in epilepsy. But breakthrough seizures happen when there is a provocation like sleep deprivation, hunger, stress, emotional outbursts, or fever. Controlling these preventable seizure triggers could help in alleviating the huge seizure burden. Patient education about proper sleep and food habits is important, especially about observance of fast, which is a common phenomenon in Indian culture. Prompt lowering down of fever with antipyretic and not missing the ASM during concurrent illness must be emphasized. Use of concomitant drugs that are potentially seizure-provoking should be checked and either eliminated or replaced with safer alternative (antibiotics, bupropion, and tramadol).

Ensure compliance: Another important factor is poor compliance to drugs. Low compliance is a common cause of treatment failure and is due to multiple contributing factors[29,30] such as (i) inadequate communication with healthcare providers, (ii) side effects of antiseizure drugs, (iii) forgetfulness,[31] and (iv) low motivation. Compliance can be improved by giving drugs at longer intervals by using either long-acting or extended-release preparations, by reminders, more frequent physician visits, and medication charts or pill counting. Documented assessment and treatment planning involving themselves and their families, inquiry and discussion about ASM side effects, and bedside testing for cognitive difficulty and then measures such as cognitive rehabilitation and family involvement are important things to ensure compliance.

■ NONPHARMACOLOGICAL TREATMENT

Role of diet is increasingly being recognized in the management of DRE, more in pediatric as compared to adult cases. In 1921, Wilder had proposed the KD as a treatment for epilepsy. The aim of the dietary therapy is to mimic starvation, as studies in the past have shown antiseizure effects under such conditions.[32] The diet encourages the intake of excessive amounts of fat and proposes daily meals containing 80% fat, 15% protein, and 5% carbohydrates. This is the so-called 4:1 (fat:nonfat) diet.[33] KD is used in the management of epileptic encephalopathies with good results. A modified diet can result in seizure freedom in 13% of patients and a reduction of >50% in seizure frequency in 53% of patients.[34] It is the first-line treatment in GLUT1 and pyruvate dehydrogenase deficiency. Modified Atkin's diet is another alternative with more tolerability. It has also been adapted as per Indian food patterns and formulas are available.[35] The major issues with diet modifications are acceptance, palatability, availability, and cost. Side effects include mainly gastrointestinal (vomiting, diarrhea, and constipation), hyperlipidemia, hypoglycemia, kidney stones, acute pancreatitis, and cardiomyopathy.

MANAGEMENT OF COMORBIDITIES

Pharmacotherapy of DREs is not restricted to the reduction of seizure burden but should include improvement of patient's QOL by providing global healthcare to the patient, which includes control of comorbidities, psychosocial support, and control of drug-related adverse events. The prevalence of comorbidities in patients with epilepsy is 2–8 times that in the general population, and about 50% of patients with epilepsy have at least one comorbidity, which is even higher in patients with DRE.[36] Stress or concurrent psychiatric illnesses must be addressed as they are shown to adversely affect seizure outcome and also influence overall QOL. Comorbid mental illness increases the risk of failing second ASM treatment.[37] Stress-management techniques including mindfulness, meditation, yoga, physical exercises can improve seizure outcomes.[38] As many as 30% patients have significant psychiatric comorbidity, which must be screened and a formal psychiatric reference should be made if required. Sleep disorder screening is not incorporated into standard epilepsy care. However, inadequate sleep is a known trigger of breakthrough seizures, and untreated sleep disorders can lower the seizure threshold.[39,40] Obstructive sleep apnea occurs in 30% of patients with epilepsy, a higher proportion than in the general population. In a pilot clinical trial, a 50% or greater reduction in seizures was observed in 28% of subjects in the therapeutic group, compared with 15% of those in the sham group.[41]

Role of dedicated epilepsy unit: Management of these drug-resistant cases requires expertise, time, and patient participation. Dedicated epilepsy clinics under care of a neurologist specializing in epilepsy services are best for management of these cases as routine busy OPDs may miss the many factors discussed earlier.[42]

CONCLUSION

In conclusion, pharmacotherapy of epilepsy has become more diversified and sophisticated by introduction of many new antiepileptic drugs (AEDs) with diverse mechanism of actions, better pharmacokinetic profiles, and better tolerability profiles, which are instrumental for the concept of patient-tailored pharmacotherapy. Rational polytherapy based on evidence can significantly increase the chances of seizure remission. Additionally, preventing seizure triggers, dietary modifications, and treating comorbidities cannot be overemphasized. The ultimate goal may not always be absolute seizure freedom in these difficult-to-manage cases but improve overall QOL by a holistic approach. Continuing trials of different rational polytherapy regimens will help to improve the outcome of the core population of epilepsy patients in the long term.

REFERENCES

1. Kwan P, Arzimanoglou A, Berg AT, Brodie MJ, Allen Hauser W, Mathern G, et al. Definition of drug resistant epilepsy: Consensus proposal by the ad hoc task force of the ILAE Commission on Therapeutic Strategies. Epilepsia. 2010;51(6): 1069-77.
2. Chen Z, Brodie MJ, Liew D, Kwan P. Treatment outcomes in patients with newly diagnosed epilepsy treated with established and new antiepileptic drugs: A 30-year longitudinal cohort study. JAMA Neurol. 2018;75(3):279-86.
3. Laxer KD, Trinka E, Hirsch LJ, Cendes F, Langfitt J, Delanty N, et al. The consequences of refractory epilepsy and its treatment. Epilepsy Behav. 2014;37:59-70.
4. Constantinescu I, Korff CM, Vulliemoz S, Picard F, Seeck M. Drug-level monitoring on admission for presurgical epilepsy evaluation. Eur Neurol. 2017;78(1-2):105-10.
5. Brodie MJ, Barry SJE, Bamagous G, Norrie JD, Kwan P. Patterns of treatment response in newly diagnosed epilepsy. Neurology. 2012;78(20): 1548-54.
6. Mula M, Zaccara G, Galimberti CA, Ferrò B, Canevini MP, Mascia A, et al. Validated outcome of treatment changes according to International League Against Epilepsy criteria in adults with drug-resistant focal epilepsy. Epilepsia 2019;60(6):1114-23.
7. Park KM, Kim SE, Lee BI. Antipeileptic drug therapy in patients with drug-resistant epilepsy. J Epilepsy Res. 2019;9(1):14-26.
8. Chi X, Li R, Hao X, Chen J, Xiong W, Xu H, et al. Response to treatment schedules after the first antiepileptic drug failed. Epilepsia. 2018;59(11):2118-24.
9. Luciano AL, Shorvon SD. Results of treatment changes in patients with apparently drug-resistant chronic epilepsy. Ann Neurol. 2007;62(4):375-81.
10. Canevini MP, De Sarro G, Galimberti CA, Gatti G, Licchetta L, Malerba A, et al. Relationship between adverse effects of antiepileptic drugs, number of coprescribed drugs, and drug load in a large cohort of consecutive patients with drug-refractory epilepsy. Epilepsia. 2010;51(5):797-804.
11. Deckers CL, Hekster YA, Keyser A, Meinardi H, Renier WO. Reappraisal of polytherapy in epilepsy: A critical review of drug load and adverse effects. Epilepsia. 1997;38(5):570-5.
12. Lammers MW, Hekster YA, Keyser A, Meinardi H, Renier WO, van Lier H. Monotherapy or polytherapy for epilepsy revisited: A quantitative assessment. Epilepsia. 1995;36(5):440-6.
13. Stephen LJ, Brodie MJ. Antiepileptic drug monotherapy versus polytherapy: Pursuing seizure freedom and tolerability in adults. Curr Opin Neurol. 2012;25(2):164-72.
14. Seiden LG, Connor GS. The importance of drug titration in the management of patients with epilepsy. Epilepsy Behav. 2022;128:108517.
15. Brodie MJ, Yuen AW. Lamotrigine substitution study: Evidence for synergism with sodium valproate? 105 study group. Epilepsy Res. 1997;26(3):423-32.
16. Kanner AM, Ashman E, Gloss D, Harden C, Bourgeois B, Bautista JF, et al. Practice guideline update summary: Efficacy and tolerability of the new antiepileptic drugs II: Treatment-resistant epilepsy. Report of the Guideline Development, Dissemination, and Implementation Sub-committee of the American Academy of Neurology and the American Epilepsy Society. Neurology. 2018;91(2):82-90.
17. Verrotti A, Lattanzi S, Brigo F, Zaccara G. Pharmacodynamic interactions of antiepileptic drugs: From bench to clinical practice. Epilepsy Behav. 2020;104:106939.
18. Brigo F, Ausserer H, Tezzon F, Nardone R. When one plus one makes three: The quest for rational antiepileptic polytherapy with supraadditive anticonvulsant efficacy. Epilepsy Behav. 2013; 27(3):439-42.
19. Sake JK, Hebert D, IsojärviJ, Doty P, De Backer M, Davies K, et al. A pooled analysis of lacosamide clinical trial data grouped by mechanism of action of concomitant antiepileptic drugs. CNS Drugs. 2010;24(12):1055-68.
20. Margolis JM, Chu BC, Wang ZJ, Copher R, Cavazos JE, et al. Effectiveness of antiepileptic drug combination therapy for partial-onset seizures based on mechanisms of action. JAMA Neurol. 2014;71(8):985-93.
21. Poolos NP, Warner LN, Humphreys SZ, Williams S. Comparative efficacy of combination drug therapy in refractory epilepsy. Neurology. 2012;78(1):62-8.
22. Khan S, Nobili L, Khatami R, Loddenkemper T, Cajochen C, Dijk DJ, et al. Circadian rhythm and epilepsy. Lancet Neurol. 2018;17(12):1098-108.
23. Nabbout R, Kuchenbuch M. Impact of predictive, preventive and precision medicine strategies in epilepsy. Nat Rev Neurol. 2020;16(12):674-88.

24. Sharma R, Nakamura M, Neupane C, Jeon BH, Shin H, Melnick SM, et al. Positive allosteric modulation of GABA$_A$ receptors by a novel antiepileptic drug cenobamate. Eur J Pharmacol. 2020;879:173117.
25. Falcicchio G, Lattanzi S, Negri F, de Tommaso M, La Neve A, Specchio N. Treatment with Cenobamate in adult patients with Lennox-Gastaut syndrome: A case series. J Clin Med. 2022;12(1):129.
26. Makridis KL, Friedo AL, Kellinghaus C, Losch FP, Schmitz B, Boßelmann C, et al. Successful treatment of adult Dravet syndrome patients with cenobamate. Epilepsia. 2022;63(12):e164-71.
27. Dini G, Tulli E, Dell'Isola GB, Mencaroni E, Di Cara G, Striano P, et al. Improving therapy of pharmacoresistant epilepsies: The role of fenfluramine. Front Pharmacol. 2022;13:832929.
28. Ji ZY, Huang YQ, He WZ. Sodium valproate combined with topiramate vs. sodium valproate alone for refractory epilepsy: A systematic review and meta-analysis. Front Neurol. 2022;12:794856.
29. Rikir E, Grisar T, Sadzot B. Le défaut d'observance thérapeutique du patient souffrant d'épilepsie. Un problème fréquent et complexe Rev Med Liège. 2010;65:366-9.
30. Malek N, Heath CA, Greene J. A review of medication adherence in people with epilepsy. Acta Neurol Scand. 2017;135(5):507-15.
31. Gurumurthy R, Chanda K, Sarma GRK. An evaluation of factors affecting adherence to antiepileptic drugs in patients with epilepsy: A cross-sectional study. Singapore Med J. 2017;58(2):98-102.
32. Mady MA, Kossoff EH, McGregor AL, Wheless JW, Pyzik PL, Freeman JM. The ketogenic diet: Adolescents can do it, too. Epilepsia. 2003;44(6):847-51.
33. Kossoff HE. More fat and fewer seizures: Dietary therapies for epilepsy. Lancet Neurol. 2004;3(7):415-20.
34. Liu H, Yang Y, Wang Y, Tang H, Zhang F, Zhang Y, et al. Ketogenic diet for treatment of intractable epilepsy in adults: A meta-analysis of observational studies. Epilepsia Open. 2018;3(1):9-17.
35. Sondhi V, Agarwala A, Pandey RM, Chakrabarty B, Jauhari P, Lodha R, et al. Efficacy of ketogenic diet, modified Atkins Diet, and Low glycemic index therapy diet among children with drug-resistant epilepsy: A Randomized clinical trial. JAMA Pediatr. 2020;174(10):944-51.
36. Keezer MR, Sisodiya SM, Sander JW. Comorbidities of epilepsy: Current concepts and future perspectives. Lancet Neurol. 2016;15(1):106-15.
37. Hatoum HT, Arcona S, Mao J, Walton S. Real-world antiseizure medication treatment outcomes in drug-resistant focal epilepsy patients. Epilepsia Open. 2023;8(4):1556-65.
38. Dawit S, Crepeau AZ. When drugs do not work: Alternatives to Antiseizure Medications. Curr Neurol Neurosci Rep. 2020;20(9):37.
39. Foldvary-Schaefer N, Andrews ND, Pornsriniyom D, Moul DE, Sun Z, Bena J. Sleep apnea and epilepsy: Who's at risk? Epilepsy Behav. 2012;25(3):363-7.
40. Lin Z, Qi Si Q, Xiaoyi Z. Obstructive sleep apnea in patients with epilepsy: A meta-analysis. Sleep Breath. 2017;21(2):263-70.
41. Malow B, Foldvary-Shafer N, Vaughn BV, Selwa LM, Chervin RD, Weatherwax KJ, et al. Treating obstructive sleep apnea in adults with epilepsy. Neurology. 2008;71(8):572-7.
42. Santulli L, Coppola A, Balestrini S, Striano S. The challenges of treating epilepsy with 25 antiepileptic drugs. Pharmacol Res. 2016;107:211-9.

CHAPTER 6

Withdrawing Antiseizure Medicines in Seizure Free Patients: Challenges and Solutions

Chaturbhuj Rathore

ABSTRACT

Withdrawal of antiseizure medicines (ASMs) in seizure-free patients poses unique challenges. The benefits of discontinuing ASMs need to be balanced with potential risks including seizure recurrence, potential loss of seizure control, and loss of sense of cure in otherwise seizure-free patients. Epilepsy being a heterogeneous disorder, a uniform approach cannot be applied while contemplating ASM withdrawal and multifactorial consideration is required to assess the chances of successful withdrawal. Only few epilepsy syndromes have well-defined prognosis following ASM withdrawal while majority of the patients have undetermined prognosis. Overall, one should consider ASM withdrawal in patients who are seizure free for >2 years. On attempted withdrawal, seizure recurrence occurs in 30–40% of the patients. The risk of seizure recurrence can be minimized with the proper selection of the patients. Patients with intellectual disability, neurological deficit, structural abnormality on magnetic resonance imaging (MRI), receiving more than one ASM, and who has had difficulty in achieving remission have a higher risk of seizure recurrence on attempted withdrawal. In such patients, withdrawal should be attempted with caution and after 5 years of seizure freedom. It is heartening to note that early or late withdrawal does not affect the natural history of epilepsy and does not lead to uncontrolled epilepsy later on. ASMs can be withdrawn in 50% of the patients after temporal lobe surgery and in 30% of the patients after extra-temporal surgeries. Various prediction models have been developed to predict the chances of successful withdrawal and serves as useful tool in practice. Patient's perspective and social circumstances are equally important while contemplating ASM withdrawal and patients should be encouraged to make an informed decision regarding ASM withdrawal.

Keywords: Antiseizure medicine, Medicine withdrawal, Epilepsy remission.

■ INTRODUCTION

All epilepsy patients receiving antiseizure medicines (ASMs) desire to stop using them. Stopping ASMs provides several benefits, including a sense of well-being and full cure for patients, a reduction in financial burden, the elimination of potential drug interactions, and cognitive, teratogenic, and other negative effects of ASMs. However, these advantages must be weighed against the possible medical and social risks, which include the possibility of having uncontrolled epilepsy in a patient whose seizures are presently controlled with

ASMs, as well as the loss of driving privileges and perception of cure following a seizure recurrence. Owing to these possible issues with ASM discontinuation and the lack of clear guidelines, clinicians remain uncertain and divided regarding ASM withdrawal in seizure free patients.[1-3]

The risk of seizure recurrence after discontinuing ASMs depends on various factors, necessitating a multifactorial consideration before making such a decision. Despite the abundance of data, predicting the precise outcome for an individual patient after ASM withdrawal remains uncertain. Therefore, it is essential to discuss all the advantages and disadvantages of ASM withdrawal with the patient to allow them to make an informed decision. Patients often have numerous questions **(Box 1)** when considering ASM withdrawal, and physicians should be able to answer these based on the available evidence, guiding the patient toward a well-informed and rational choice. This review aims to address the challenges encountered when considering ASM withdrawal in seizure-free patients and offers practical solutions and tips.

■ PRACTICAL CONSIDERATION BEFORE ANTISEIZURE MEDICINE WITHDRAWAL

Physicians should weigh the risks and benefits before contemplating ASM withdrawal in seizure free patients. The most important factor that needs to be considered is the risk of seizure recurrence on attempted withdrawal. Similarly, a small proportion of patients also have a risk of loss of seizure control once they have seizure recurrence during or after ASM discontinuation. The risk of seizure recurrence is determined by multiple factors and is difficult to predict in individual patients. The most important factor which determine the risk of recurrence is the underlying epilepsy syndrome. However, only few epilepsy syndromes have well-defined prognosis with regard to ASM withdrawal **(Table 1)**. Patients with benign focal epilepsies have low risk of seizure recurrence and ASMs can be safely withdrawn in these patients after a reasonable period of seizure freedom. On the other hand, it is difficult to withdraw ASMs in patients with juvenile myoclonic

BOX 1: Common concerns of epilepsy patients regarding antiseizure medicine (ASM) withdrawal.

- How long I need to continue my medicines?
- When can we stop ASMs?
- Will I again have a seizure after ASM withdrawal?
- What are the chances of having a seizure after ASM withdrawal?
- In case of a recurrence, whether my seizures will be again controlled?
- Are there any other major risks after withdrawal, e.g., status epilepticus?
- Over how many days/months my medicines will be reduced?
- Would I be able to drive during and after ASM withdrawal?

TABLE 1: Probabilities of successful antiseizure medicine withdrawal in various epilepsy syndromes.

Syndromes	Successful withdrawal
Benign rolandic epilepsy, benign occipital epilepsy	95–100%
Childhood absence epilepsy	80%
Genetic generalized epilepsy (unclassified)	60%
Cryptogenic focal epilepsy	60–70%
Juvenile absence epilepsy, Juvenile myoclonic epilepsy	10–30%
Epileptic encephalopathies, Rasmussen's encephalitis, Reading epilepsy	0–5%

epilepsy (JME), who have a higher risk of seizure recurrence on attempted withdrawal. However, the vast majority of the patients fall in between these extremes and have syndromes with intermediate prognosis. It is difficult to predict precise outcome in such patients and careful assessment of pros and cons of ASM withdrawal is required in these patients. The other important factors which merit consideration before contemplating ASM withdrawal are duration of seizure freedom, number of ASMs being used, and the presence of epileptiform abnormalities on electroencephalogram (EEG).

■ RISK OF SEIZURE RECURRENCE ON ANTISEIZURE MEDICINE WITHDRAWAL

As discussed earlier, it is difficult to precisely determine the risk of seizure recurrence in an individual patient. The available studies and data do provide some broad guidelines. However, the majority of these studies are nonrandomized observational studies, which have included heterogeneous groups of patients, and thus preclude any definite conclusions. Even in randomized studies, there is no ideal control group as it is not possible to continue ASMs indefinitely, which makes it difficult to assess the risk of seizure recurrence while being continued on ASMs.

Only two randomized trials have documented the risk of seizure recurrence after withdrawal of ASMs, with patients randomly assigned to either continued treatment or gradual ASM withdrawal. The first and largest prospective randomized, nonblinded study was conducted by the Medical Research Council (MRC) Antiepileptic Drug Withdrawal Group.[4] In this study, 1,013 patients who had been seizure-free for at least 2 years were randomly allocated to continue taking ASMs or undergo gradual withdrawal over 6 months. Participants in the continued-treatment group were given the option of ASM withdrawal after 2 years. At 2 years, the relapse rate was 22% in the continued-treatment group compared to 41% in the withdrawal group. This study reflected a real-world clinical setting and included a diverse group of patients meeting the sole criterion of being seizure-free for at least 2 years. Notably, 15% of patients had developmental delay and 20% had some form of neurological impairment.

The Akershus study was a truly randomized double-blind trial in which 160 patients who had been seizure-free for over 2 years on ASM monotherapy were randomly divided into two groups: ASM withdrawal (n = 79) and nonwithdrawal (n = 81).[5] The study had strict eligibility criteria and excluded patients on more than one ASMs, patients with JME, patients of genetic generalized epilepsy with abnormal EEG, and individuals with intellectual disabilities. Follow-up evaluations were conducted in a double-blind manner for up to 12 months or until seizure recurrence. After 1 year, seizure relapse rates were 15% in the withdrawal group, and 7% in the nonwithdrawal group [relative risk (RR) 2.46; 95% confidence interval (CI) 0.85–7.08; p = 0.095]. Subsequently, patients from the nonwithdrawal group entered an open withdrawal phase after 1 year and were monitored for an average of 47 months. In this open follow-up, 27% of the patients experienced seizure recurrence. The lower relapse rates in this study can be partly attributed to the stringent selection criteria, which excluded patients with a higher risk of relapse. This study suggests that meticulous patient selection can reduce the risk of recurrence.

In addition to these specific controlled trials, numerous other observational studies, meta-analyses, systematic reviews, and practice guidelines have been published on this subject.[6-8] Collectively, these data indicate that, on average, the rate of seizure recurrence after 2 years of ASM discontinuation in unselected patients is around 30% for children and 40% for adults. A recent meta-analysis encompassing 45 studies revealed that the risk of relapse following ASM discontinuation was 22% (95% CI 19–26%) at 1 year, 28% (24–32%) at 2 years, and 34% (28–40%) at 3 or 4 years.[8] Recurrences after 5 years were observed in only 1% of the patients. Overall, discontinuing ASMs increases the immediate risk of seizure recurrence by two-fold, although this risk can be mitigated through careful patient selection.

■ PREDICTORS OF RELAPSE AFTER ANTISEIZURE MEDICINE WITHDRAWAL

Understanding the factors that help in predicting seizure recurrence after discontinuing ASMs is crucial for selecting appropriate candidates for withdrawal and estimating the personalized risk of relapse. In spite of limitations in predating the risk of relapse in individual patients, certain general conclusions can be drawn from existing research and clinical experience.

In a systematic review of 45 articles focusing on predictors of seizure relapse after ASM withdrawal, Lamberink and colleagues identified a total of 25 distinct predictors.[8] However, they also highlighted the lack of consistency among these predictors, with many showing conflicting results across studies. They also noted the overall low quality of many studies and significant variability in study populations. Despite these challenges, certain factors have consistently emerged as reliable predictors of outcome following ASM withdrawal **(Box 2)**. The main factors that are strongly associated with an increased risk of seizure recurrence include symptomatic etiology, presence of structural abnormality on magnetic resonance imaging (MRI), presence of neurological deficits or cognitive

> **BOX 2: Factors associated with a higher risk of seizure recurrence on ASM withdrawal in medically-treated patients.**
>
> - Neurological deficit
> - Intellectual disability
> - Structural abnormality on MRI
> - Higher number of seizures before remission (difficult initial control)
> - History of seizures while on ASM therapy (difficult initial control)
> - Shorter period of remission (<2 years)
> - Abnormal EEG (prior to or during ASM withdrawal)
> - Focal epilepsy
> - Multiple seizure types
> - Myoclonic seizures
> - Neonatal or complex febrile seizures
> - Receiving more than one drug at the time of withdrawal
> - Adolescent or adult age at epilepsy onset
>
> (ASM: antiseizure medicine; EEG: electroencephalogram; MRI: magnetic resonance imaging)

impairment, and difficulty in the initial control of epilepsy.[9-12] Additionally, the presence of definite epileptiform abnormalities on EEG, either before or during withdrawal, increases the likelihood of relapse following ASM cessation.[13,14] However, making a decision based solely on EEG findings may not be appropriate, as certain epilepsies such as benign rolandic epilepsy can have abnormal EEG long after seizure remission. While undertaking an EEG prior to considering ASM withdrawal is a standard practice, the decision should not be based on EEG findings alone.

The duration from treatment initiation to achieving seizure control also serves as a significant predictor of relapse. Longer duration in attaining seizure freedom and the use of more than one ASMs indicate difficult initial control of epilepsy and correlate with a higher risk of relapse after

ASM withdrawal.[5,10,11] Similarly, a greater number of seizures (10 or more) before achieving remission is also linked to a higher risk of recurrence following ASM withdrawal.[11]

PREDICTION MODELS FOR SEIZURE RECURRENCE ON ANTISEIZURE MEDICINE WITHDRAWAL

Numerous researchers have tried to construct models for predicting the risk of seizure recurrence after ASM withdrawal in individual patients **(Table 2)**.[11,15-19]

These models integrate various predictors to estimate the risk of relapse for a specific patient. Overall, these models offer moderate predictive capability and serve as an important tool to aid in the decision-making process regarding ASM withdrawal.

One such model, known as the MRC prognostic index, was developed by the MRC antiepileptic drug withdrawal group and validated on a large cohort.[16] This model consisting of seven factors is designed to predict the risk of seizure recurrence at 1 and 2 years after ASM withdrawal. In the validation cohort, the calculated probabilities closely matched with the actual recurrence

TABLE 2: Various prediction models for seizure relapse on antiseizure medicine (ASM) withdrawal.*

References	Study characteristics	Patient numbers	Included variables
Overweg et al., 1987[15]	Adults, seizure free for >3 years	62	• Number of ASMs • Serum level of ASMs • Age at last seizure • Duration of seizure-freedom
MRC prognostic index, 1993[16]	Unselected adults and children	1,003	• Age ≥16 years • Use of more than one ASM • Seizures after starting ASM • Presence of tonic-clonic seizures • Myoclonic seizures • Abnormal EEG • Duration of seizure freedom
Dooley et al., 1995[17]	Children, seizure free for >1 year	97	• Female sex • Age at seizure onset • Seizure (generalized versus partial) • Neurological abnormalities
Braathen and Melander, 1997[18]	Children, seizure free for >1 year	161	• Seizure type and epilepsy type • Age at onset • Type of EEG abnormality
Geerts et al., 2005[19]	Children, seizure free for >6 months	161	• Age at onset of epilepsy • Absence etiology • Idiopathic etiology • Abnormal EEG • Postictal signs

Continued

Continued

References	Study characteristics	Patient numbers	Included variables
Lamberink et al., 2017[11]	Adults and children	1,769	• Duration of epilepsy • Duration of seizure freedom • Febrile seizures • Age at onset of epilepsy • Number of seizures before remission • Absence of a self-limiting syndrome • Developmental delay • Epileptiform abnormalities on EEG
Lamberink et al., 2018[39]	Children following epilepsy surgery	766	• Age at withdrawal • Timing of ASM withdrawal following surgery • Multifocal MRI abnormalities • Abnormal postoperative EEG • Incomplete resection
Rathore et al., 2018 (FND20 score)[34]	Adults and children following temporal lobectomy	384	• Febrile seizures • Normal postoperative EEG • Duration of epilepsy

*Almost all the models have predictive value of 60–70%.

rates. Despite its robustness, the model is somewhat complicated and challenging to implement in clinical settings.

More recently, Lamberink and colleagues developed a model to predict the risk of seizure recurrence and long-term outcomes subsequent to ASM withdrawal through a meta-analysis of individual patient data from 10 studies encompassing 1,769 patients.[11] Through a multivariate analysis, they identified eight factors linked with the risk of seizure relapse after ASM withdrawal **(Table 2)**. Using these factors, the authors developed nomograms and an online tool to forecast the probability of seizure recurrence post-ASM withdrawal and the likelihood of experiencing seizures in the final year of follow-up. Both models exhibited strong performance, with adjusted concordance statistics reaching 0.65 for predicting seizure recurrence and 0.71 for forecasting long-term seizure freedom. The calculator based on these models can be accessed at https://tinyurl.com/uxyu26p (www. http://epilepsypredictiontools.info), enabling users to estimate the risk of seizure recurrence at 2- and 5-year after ASM withdrawal, along with the probability of seizure freedom a decade after withdrawal. This calculator is easy to use and very useful tool for clinical decision making. However, all these models possess only a moderate predictive capacity, indicating that the outcomes after ASM withdrawal depend upon multiple factors, and it is challenging to precisely predict individual patient outcomes in a condition as diverse as epilepsy.

■ TIMING AND SPEED OF ANTISEIZURE MEDICINE WITHDRAWAL

Duration of seizure freedom before considering ASM withdrawal is an important predictor of seizure relapse. A longer duration of seizure freedom is more likely to be associated with epilepsy remission and a higher chance of successful ASM withdrawal.[6,7,11,16] The MRC study indicated that a seizure freedom of 5 years or more was associated with a lower risk of recurrence as compared to a seizure freedom of <2.5 years.[4,16] Similarly, a Cochrane review suggested that patients with seizure freedom of <2 years had a higher risk of recurrence on attempted withdrawal, as compared to those with a seizure freedom of >2 years.[20] In the early withdrawal study in children where withdrawal was attempted after 6 months of seizure freedom, recurrence rate was as high as 50%.[21] Thus, overall data indicate that in unselected group of patients, a seizure freedom of at least 2 years is ideal before considering ASM withdrawal. Adults have a higher risk of seizure recurrence as compared to children, and hence a longer period of seizure freedom of 3–4 years may be more suitable in adults before contemplating ASM withdrawal.[8,22] We usually consider ASM withdrawal after 2 years of seizure freedom in children and after 4 years of seizure freedom in adults. However, the early withdrawal and subsequent recurrence do not affect the long-term outcome of epilepsy and only indicate that epilepsy is still active at the time of withdrawal.

If one decides to withdraw ASMs, then next consideration is the process and rate of withdrawal. The overall data with regard to rate of ASM withdrawal is inconclusive leading to variable practices. The question of rate of withdrawal has been studied in 10 studies, almost exclusively in children.[23] In a randomized trial, involving 149 children, rapid withdrawal over 6 weeks was associated with a marginally higher recurrence risk as compared to slow withdrawal over 9 months.[24] Other nonrandomized studies have also suggested that a rapid withdrawal over 1 month is associated with a higher risk of relapse.[23,25,26] In view of this data, we usually withdraw one ASM over a period of 3–4 months. The withdrawal rate should be even slower with medicines having higher risk of withdrawal seizures such as phenobarbitone and clobazam, and we taper these medicines over 6 months.

There are no definite guidelines regarding ASM withdrawal in patients receiving more than one medicines. Most studies on ASM withdrawal have included all patients, regardless of the number of medications they are on. These patients often have initially difficult-to-control epilepsy and have a higher risk of recurrence after withdrawal.[8,11] These patients also have a higher risk of uncontrolled epilepsy after recurrence on attempted withdrawal. In these patients, we typically start withdrawal after 5 years of seizure freedom and withdraw one drug at a time with a period of 12 months between the withdrawal of two medicines.

■ TIMING OF SEIZURE RECURRENCE ON ANTISEIZURE MEDICINE WITHDRAWAL

The majority of the seizure recurrences on attempted ASM withdrawal occur within 1 year of discontinuation. In a meta-analysis focusing on risk of relapse following ASM withdrawal, two-thirds of the recurrences occurred within 1 year of discontinuation, while only 6% of the patients had seizure recurrence after 2 years of discontinuation.[8] Similarly, the long-term follow-up of MRC cohort showed that 1 year risk of relapse at 0, 3, 6, and 12 months following withdrawal is 30%, 15%, 9%, and 9%, respectively, suggesting that risk after 6 months of withdrawal is sufficiently low.[27] These data have important implications for counseling the patients regarding driving during the process of ASM withdrawal. The United Kingdom guidelines prohibit patients to drive during ASM withdrawal and for a period of 6 months after discontinuation. In case of seizure recurrence after ASM discontinuation, the 1-year risk of subsequent seizures after restarting medicines is 26% at 3 months and 18% at 6 months.[27] European Union guidelines permit patients to resume driving 3 months after restarting ASMs, whereas United Kingdom guidelines require a 1-year period before driving can be resumed after restarting medication.

■ RISK OF UNCONTROLLED EPILEPSY AFTER ANTISEIZURE MEDICINE WITHDRAWAL

The most important consideration before contemplating ASM withdrawal is the risk of uncontrolled seizures after ASM withdrawal. A few observational studies and a systematic review have indicated that approximately 15-20% of patients do not regain seizure control once seizures recur following ASM withdrawal.[28] This data creates significant hesitation among clinicians when considering ASM withdrawal. However, majority of the other studies have suggested a very low risk of uncontrolled epilepsy following ASM discontinuation. In a population-based and a long-term follow-up study involving 260 children, only three (1%) had developed uncontrolled epilepsy after ASM discontinuation.[29] Similarly, long-term follow-up of patients in MRC study has shown that 95% of patients achieve 1 year seizure freedom after restarting ASMs.[10] The MRC data also suggest that long-term seizure control is similar in patients who undergo early or late ASM withdrawal. Thus, ASM withdrawal does not alter the natural history of epilepsy. Similarly, there is no increased risk of status epilepticus or sudden unexplained death in epilepsy (SUDEP) in those patients who undergo ASM withdrawal.[30] These data are reassuring and suggest that the risk of uncontrolled epilepsy after ASM discontinuation in majority of the patients is low. However, patients with structural etiology, cognitive impairment, and a history of difficulty in controlling epilepsy initially have a higher risk of uncontrolled seizures after ASM discontinuation.[28] Therefore, caution should be exercised when considering ASM withdrawal for these patients, and a thorough discussion of the risks and benefits should be undertaken with the patient.

■ ANTISEIZURE MEDICINE WITHDRAWAL FOLLOWING EPILEPSY SURGERY

One of the most important objectives of the patients undergoing epilepsy surgery is to discontinue ASMs.[31] As compared to medically treated patients, there is a relative dearth of data regarding ASM withdrawal after epilepsy surgery. There has been no randomized controlled trial of ASM withdrawal in patients undergoing epilepsy surgery and the data largely comes from few observational studies. Still, few practical conclusions can be drawn.

The success of ASM withdrawal depends upon the type of epilepsy surgery. In patients undergoing anterior temporal lobectomy for mesial temporal lobe epilepsy, ASM withdrawal can be attempted in 70% of the patients. Antiseizure medicines can be stopped in approximately 50% of the patients at 3 years following surgery.[32,33] Seizure recurrence usually occurs in 25% of the patients on attempted withdrawal, of which >90% again become seizure free after restarting ASM.[33,34] In patients with extra-temporal surgeries, ASM can be discontinued in 25-30% of the patients at 3 years of follow-up.[35-37] These patients also have a higher risk of seizure recurrence on attempted withdrawal which occurs on 30-50% of the patients.

Certain important predictors of successful ASM withdrawal have been identified in patients who undergo epilepsy surgery **(Box 3)**. In patients undergoing temporal lobectomy, preoperative epilepsy duration of >20 years, absence of febrile seizures, abnormal EEG at 1 year following surgery, and absence of hippocampal sclerosis on pathology are associated with a lower chance of successful ASM withdrawal.[33,34,38] In extra-temporal surgeries, the factors associated with an increased risk of recurrence on ASM withdrawal are: Longer preoperative epilepsy duration, presence of interictal epileptiform discharges on postoperative EEG, early postoperative seizures, incomplete resection of the lesion, multifocal MRI abnormalities, and presence of gliosis or dysplasia on MRI.[35-37] Based on these predictors, two prediction models have been developed to predict the individualized risk of seizure recurrence on ASM withdrawal in postoperative patients. Based on TimetoStop cohort of 766 children, Lamberink and colleagues prepared nomogram and a model to predict the individualized risk of 2- and 5-year recurrence on ASM withdrawal and seizure freedom at the last follow-up.[39] The web-based tool is available at: https://tinyurl.com/wptmz3t (http://www.epilepsypredictiontools.info/ttswithdrawal) and is useful for predicting individualized risk of seizure recurrence on attempted withdrawal. Internal-external cross-validation shows a concordance statistic of 0.68 for predicting recurrence risk and 0.73 for predicting seizure free outcome at last follow-up. In our study of 384 patients, who have undergone temporal lobectomy, epilepsy duration of >20 years, absence of febrile seizures, and interictal epileptiform discharges on 1-year postoperative EEG were significant predictors of seizure recurrence on ASM withdrawal on multivariate analysis.[34] Based upon these three factors we developed FND20 score (febrile seizures, normal EEG at 1 year, duration <20 years) to predict the risk of seizure recurrence on ASM withdrawal. When all the three factors are favorable (FND20 score = 3), the chance of recurrence is 17%, while it is 59% if all the three factors are unfavorable (FND20 = 0). The score has very good negative predictive value and a modest positive predictive value for predicting seizure recurrence and is useful for identifying ideal candidates for ASM withdrawal. We also calculated the chances of complete ASM discontinuation in the cohort and found five factors predictive of complete ASM discontinuation at the last follow-up. We formulated No-FUNDS score (no febrile seizures, no unilateral interictal discharges on preoperative EEG, no normal postoperative EEG, no duration <20 years, and no sclerosis on MRI; **Box 4**). These three models can be used to predict the chances of seizure recurrence on attempted ASM withdrawal and are quite useful while counseling the patients for ASM management following epilepsy surgery.

The timing of starting ASM withdrawal after epilepsy surgery is not well defined. In Timetostop study, early withdrawal was associated with a higher risk of seizure

> **BOX 3: Factors associated with higher risk of seizure recurrence on ASM withdrawal following epilepsy surgery.**
>
> - Longer preoperative duration of epilepsy (>20 years)
> - Older age at surgery
> - Incomplete resection of MRI abnormality
> - Interictal epileptiform discharges on post-operative EEG
> - Early withdrawal following surgery
> - Absence of febrile seizures (for TLE)
> - Absence of hippocampal sclerosis on pathology (for TLE)
> - Multifocal abnormalities on preoperative MRI (for ETLE)
>
> (ASM: antiseizure medicines; EEG: electroencephalogram; ETLE: extratemporal lobe epilepsy; MRI: magnetic resonance imaging; TLE: temporal lobe epilepsy)

> **BOX 4: Ideal candidates for ASM withdrawal following temporal lobectomy.**
>
> - (F) Febrile seizures
> - (U) Unilateral interictal epileptiform discharges on preoperative EEG
> - (N) Normal postoperative EEG
> - (D) Duration of epilepsy <20 years
> - (S) Sclerosis on MRI
>
> *Note:* Absence of any one of these factors (No-FUNDS score) increases the probability of remaining on antiseizure medicines after temporal lobectomy. Absence of three factors has 93% probability of remaining on antiseizure medicines following temporal lobectomy.
>
> (ASM: antiseizure medicine; EEG: electroencephalogram; MRI: magnetic resonance imaging)

recurrence.[39] However, the final seizure freedom did not differ between patients who underwent early or late withdrawal. We found the similar results in a study of 135 patients, who had undergone anterior temporal lobectomy, and ASM withdrawal was started at 1 versus 3 years following surgery.[40] Thus, it can be summarized that early ASM withdrawal does not alter the natural history of disease but just unmasks the surgical failure. We usually start withdrawing medicines at 1 year following surgery, and discontinue by 3 years after surgery, except in patients with focal cortical dysplasia and gliosis, where we continue one ASM for 5 years. We follow a protocol of slow withdrawal of ASMs and discontinue one ASM over 6–9 months.

■ ANTISEIZURE MEDICINE WITHDRAWAL IN SPECIAL POPULATIONS

While the general principles of ASM withdrawal apply to most patients, certain groups present unique challenges that require special consideration, as discussed further.

Antiseizure Medicine Withdrawal in Elderly

Epilepsy is common in people above 60 years of age. The majority of the patients with epilepsy onset after 60 years of age have symptomatic focal epilepsy. The epilepsy is well controlled in 80–90% of elderly people. There has been no study focusing on ASM withdrawal in elderly and this population is not well represented in other studies of ASM withdrawal. Hence, the practice of ASM withdrawal in elderly patients largely depends upon anecdotal evidence and personal experience. The risk of seizure recurrence in elderly patients is undetermined but considered to be as high as 80–90%.[41] This along with the risks associated with major seizures in elderly make it difficult to withdraw ASMs. Due to these factors and the lack of definitive evidence, most experts recommend lifelong ASM treatment for elderly patients, and we adhere to this practice as well.

Antiseizure Medicine Withdrawal in Juvenile Myoclonic Epilepsy

Till recently, JME and juvenile absence epilepsy (JAE) were considered as lifelong disorders, and it was a common practice to continue ASM indefinitely in these patients. The earlier studies had shown a seizure recurrence of 80–100% in JME patients on attempted ASM withdrawal.[42,43] However, these studies included younger patients, where ASM was attempted after 3–4 years of seizure freedom. Recent long-term follow-up studies with follow-up periods ranging from 25 to 63 years in patients with JME, have shown that approximately one-third of patients can discontinue their medicines.[44,45] These studies indicate that JME is a heterogeneous disorder and all patients do not require indefinite ASMs. Antiseizure medicine withdrawal should be attempted in these patients after 40 years of age when they are seizure free for 5 years and have normal EEG.

Antiseizure Medicine Withdrawal in Neurocysticercosis

Neurocysticercosis is the most common cause of new onset focal epilepsy in Indian subcontinent and Latin America. Patients with single cysticercal granuloma have infrequent seizures which are easily controlled with ASMs. Many observational studies have suggested that ASMs can be safely withdrawn in these patients after 4–12 weeks of resolution of the lesion.[46-48] However, those patients with more than two seizures and those with residual calcified lesions have higher chance of seizure recurrence on attempted ASM withdrawal.[48] We usually continue ASMs for 5 years in patients with residual calcified lesions.

Antiseizure Medicine Withdrawal after Acute Symptomatic Seizures

Patients with seizures due to acute neurological disorders behave differently from other patients with epilepsy as these patients do not have chronic predisposition for unprovoked seizures. The recurrence risk on these patients is sufficiently low so that these patients may not be classified as having epilepsy.[49] In the absence of any reliable data or controlled trials, the ideal duration of ASM therapy in these patients is undetermined and largely guided by the clinical experience and expert guidelines. The important factor determining the duration of ASM therapy is the perceived risk of seizure recurrence which depends upon the type and severity of initial injury. In one retrospective study, the risk of unprovoked seizures at 10-year of follow-up was 30.8% for hypoxic injury, 10.8% for metabolic causes, and 23.9% for patients with other structural etiologies including stroke, traumatic brain injury, and neuro-infections.[50] For practical purposes, it is important to differentiate between patients who fully recover with no MRI abnormalities and those who have residual structural abnormalities on MRI. Patients with residual MRI lesions have a higher likelihood of recurrence and may require prolonged treatment.[51,52] In contrast, patients with fully resolved acute metabolic or toxic etiologies typically need only short-term seizure suppression or ASMs for 1-week postrecovery. Similarly, ASMs can be discontinued after a week in patients with mild-to-moderate head injury. For patients with subarachnoid hemorrhage, acute stroke, cerebral venous sinus thrombosis, and acute encephalitis with residual MRI changes, we usually maintain ASMs for 1–2 years, before considering withdrawal. If there are no structural abnormalities on MRI, we stop ASMs 3 months after the acute symptomatic seizures.

■ CONCLUSION

The key aspects of ASM withdrawal are summarized in **Box 5**. ASM withdrawal should be considered for any patient who has been seizure-free for over 2 years. Discontinuing ASMs does not increase the risk of uncontrolled epilepsy, status epilepticus, or SUDEP. The risk of relapse after ASM withdrawal ranges from 30 to 40%, but this can be minimized by carefully selecting patients and identifying ideal candidates **(Boxes 4 and 6)**. Patients with neurological deficit, intellectual disability, structural abnormalities on MRI, abnormal EEG at the time of withdrawal, and those who had difficult to control epilepsy initially have a higher risk of relapse. However, these factors should be used to delay, rather than

BOX 5: Salient features of antiseizure medicine (ASM) withdrawal in seizure-free patients.

- Only 20% patients have epilepsy syndromes with well-defined prognosis
- Majority of the patients have intermediate, uncertain prognosis following ASM withdrawal
- Approximately 30–40% of patients have recurrence on attempted ASM withdrawal
- Approximately 20% of seizure-free patients have recurrence even while on continued ASM therapy
- ASM withdrawal increases the risk of seizure relapse by two-fold as compared to continued treatment without affecting long-term prognosis
- Risk of recurrence can be minimized to 10–15% by careful selection of the patients
- Majority (~90%) of patients remain well controlled after seizure relapse
- Epilepsy may become uncontrolled in 1–5% of patients following recurrence on ASM withdrawal
- Minimum 2-year seizure freedom is appropriate before planning ASM withdrawal; longer period (3–4 years) may be preferable in adults
- Three most important predictors for relapse are symptomatic etiology, presence of neurological deficit, and initial difficult control of epilepsy
- ASM withdrawal should be attempted with caution and after 5 years of seizure freedom in patients with any of the above risk factors
- Gradual withdrawal over 3–6 months is the most appropriate protocol of withdrawal
- ASMs can be discontinued in 40–50% of the patients following temporal lobe surgery and in 25% of the patients after extra-temporal surgery
- Decision of ASM withdrawal should be individualized after proper assessment of risks and benefits and according to patient's wishes

BOX 6: Ideal candidates for ASM withdrawal on medical treatment.

- Seizure-free for ≥2 years
- Normal neurological examination
- Normal IQ
- Normal brain MRI
- Normal prewithdrawal EEG
- Early control with single ASM
- Juvenile myoclonic epilepsy excluded

(ASM: antiseizure medicine; EEG: electroencephalogram; IQ: intelligence quotient; MRI: magnetic resonance imaging)

deny, withdrawal. In these patients with one of the risk factors, we advocate considering ASM withdrawal in patients who have been seizure-free for 5 years or more. Various prediction models and online tools can help assess the individual risk of seizure relapse after ASM withdrawal and should be used routinely in clinical practice. Since epilepsy is a heterogeneous disease with variable outcomes, a one-size-fits-all approach is not appropriate for ASM withdrawal. Each case requires an individualized, informed decision in line with the patient's preferences.

REFERENCES

1. Schmidt D. AED discontinuation may be dangerous for seizure-free patients. J Neural Transm. 2011;118(2):183-6.
2. Beghi E. AED discontinuation may not be dangerous in seizure-free patients. J Neural Transm. 2011;118(2):187-91.
3. Specchio LM, Beghi E. Should antiepileptic drugs be withdrawn in seizure-free patients? CNS Drugs. 2004;18(4):201-12.
4. Medical Research Council Antiepileptic Drug Withdrawal Study Group Randomised study of antiepileptic drug withdrawal in patients in remission. Lancet. 1991;337(8751):1175-80.

5. Lossius MI, Hessen E, Mowinckel P, Stavem K, Erikssen J, Gulbrandsen P, et al. Consequences of antiepileptic drug withdrawal: a randomized, double-blind study (Akershus Study). Epilepsia. 2008;49(3):455-63.
6. Berg AT, Shinnar S. Relapse following discontinuation of antiepileptic drugs: a meta-analysis. Neurology. 1994;44(4):601-8.
7. Gloss D, Pargeon K, Pack A, Varma J, French JA, Tolchin B, et al.; AAN Guideline Subcommittee. Antiseizure Medication Withdrawal in Seizure-Free Patients: Practice Advisory Update Summary: Report of the AAN Guideline Subcommittee. Neurology. 2021;97(23):1072-81.
8. Lamberink HJ, Otte WM, Geleijns K, Braun KP. Antiepileptic drug withdrawal in medically and surgically treated patients: a meta-analysis of seizure recurrence and systematic review of its predictors. Epileptic Disord. 2015;17(3):211-28.
9. Yang W, Zhang X, Long J, Wu Q, Han Y. Prediction of the recurrence risk in patients with epilepsy after the withdrawal of antiepileptic drugs. Epilepsy Behav. 2020;110:107156.
10. Chadwick D, Taylor J, Johnson T. Outcomes after seizure recurrence in people with well-controlled epilepsy and the factors that influence it. The MRC Antiepileptic Drug Withdrawal Group. Epilepsia. 1996;37(11):1043-50.
11. Lamberink HJ, Otte WM, Geerts AT, Pavlovic M, Ramos-Lizana J, Marson AG, et al. Individualised prediction model of seizure recurrence and long-term outcomes after withdrawal of antiepileptic drugs in seizure-free patients: a systematic review and individual participant data meta-analysis. Lancet Neurol. 2017;16(7):523-31.
12. Cardoso TA, Coan AC, Kobayashi E, Guerreiro CA, Li LM, Cendes F. Hippocampal abnormalities and seizure recurrence after antiepileptic drug withdrawal. Neurology. 2006;67(1):134-6.
13. Tang L, Xiao Z. Can electroencephalograms provide guidance for the withdrawal of antiepileptic drugs: A meta-analysis. Clin Neurophysiol. 2017;128(2):297-302.
14. Yao J, Wang H, Xiao Z. Correlation between EEG during AED withdrawal and epilepsy recurrence: a meta-analysis. Neurol Sci. 2019;40(8):1637-44.
15. Overweg J, Binnie CD, Oosting J, Rowan AJ. Clinical and EEG prediction of seizure recurrence following antiepileptic drug withdrawal. Epilepsy Res. 1987;1(5):272-83.
16. Medical Research Council Antiepileptic Drug Withdrawal Study Group. Prognostic index for recurrence of seizures after remission of epilepsy. BMJ. 1993;306:1374-8.
17. Dooley J, Gordon K, Camfield P, Camfield C, Smith E. Discontinuation of anticonvulsant therapy in children free of seizures for 1 year: A prospective study. Neurology. 1996;46(4):969-74.
18. Braathen G, Melander H. Early discontinuation of treatment in children with uncomplicated epilepsy: a prospective study with a model for prediction of outcome. Epilepsia. 1997;38(5):561-9.
19. Geerts AT, Niermeijer JM, Peters AC, Arts WF, Brouwer OF, Stroink H, et al. Four-year outcome after early withdrawal of antiepileptic drugs in childhood epilepsy. Neurology. 2005;64(12):2136-8.
20. Strozzi I, Nolan SJ, Sperling MR, Wingerchuk DM, Sirven J. Early versus late antiepileptic drug withdrawal for people with epilepsy in remission. Cochrane Database Syst Rev. 2015;2:CD001902.
21. Peters AC, Brouwer OF, Geerts AT, Arts WF, Stroink H, van Donselaar CA. Randomized prospective study of early discontinuation of antiepileptic drugs in children with epilepsy. Neurology. 1998;50(3):724-30.
22. Camfield P, Camfield C. When is it safe to discontinue AED treatment? Epilepsia. 2008;49(Suppl 9):25-8.
23. Beghi E, Giussani G, Grosso S, Iudice A, La Neve A, Pisani F, et al. Withdrawal of antiepileptic drugs: Guidelines of the Italian League Against Epilepsy. Epilepsia. 2013;54(Suppl 7):2-12.
24. Tennison M, Greenwood R, Lewis D, Thorn M. Discontinuing antiepileptic drugs in children with epilepsy: a comparison of a six-week and a nine-month taper period. NEJM. 1994;330(20):1407-10.
25. Serra JG, Montenegro MA, Guerreiro MM. Antiepileptic drug withdrawal in childhood: does the duration of tapering off matter for seizure recurrence? J Child Neurol. 2005;20(7):624-6.
26. Ayuga Loro F, Gisbert Tijeras E, Brigo F. Rapid versus slow withdrawal of antiepileptic drugs. Cochrane Database Syst Rev. 2020;1(1):CD005003.
27. Bonnett LJ, Shukralla A, Tudur-Smith C, Williamson PR, Marson AG. Seizure recurrence after antiepileptic drug withdrawal and the implications for driving: further results from the MRC Antiepileptic Drug Withdrawal Study and a systematic review. J Neurol Neurosurg Psychiatry. 2011;82(12):1328-33.
28. Schmidt D, Löscher W. Uncontrolled epilepsy following discontinuation of antiepileptic drugs in seizure-free patients: a review of current clinical experience. Acta Neurol Scand. 2005;111(5):291-300.

29. Camfield P, Camfield C. The frequency of intractable seizures after stopping AEDs in seizure-free children with epilepsy. Neurology. 2005;64(6):973-5.
30. Camfield CS, Camfield PR, Veugelers P. Death in children with childhood onset epilepsy: a population-based study. Lancet. 2002;359(9321): 1892-5.
31. Taylor DC, McMackin D, Staunton H, Delanty N, Phillips J. Patients' aims for epilepsy surgery: desire beyond seizure freedom. Epilepsia. 2001; 42(5):629-33.
32. Schiller Y, Cascino GD, So EL, Marsh WR. Discontinuation of antiepileptic drugs after successful epilepsy surgery. Neurology. 2000; 54(2):346-9.
33. Rathore C, Panda S, Sarma PS, Radhakrishnan K. How safe is it to withdraw antiepileptic drugs following successful surgery for mesial temporal lobe epilepsy? Epilepsia. 2011;52(3):627-35.
34. Rathore C, Jeyaraj MK, Dash GK, Wattamwar P, Baheti N, Sarma SP, et al. Outcome after seizure recurrence on antiepileptic drug withdrawal following temporal lobectomy. Neurology. 2018;91(3):e208-16.
35. Park KI, Lee SK, Chu K, Jung KH, Bae EK, Kim JS, et al. Withdrawal of antiepileptic drugs after neocortical epilepsy surgery. Ann Neurol. 2010;67(2):230-38.
36. Menon R, Rathore C, Sarma SP, Radhakrishnan K. Feasibility of antiepileptic drug withdrawal following extratemporal resective epilepsy surgery. Neurology. 2012;79(8):770-6.
37. Boshuisen K, Arzimanoglou A, Cross JH, Uiterwaal CS, Polster T, van Nieuwenhuizen O, et al.; TimeToStop study group. Timing of antiepileptic drug withdrawal and long-term seizure outcome after paediatric epilepsy surgery (TimeToStop): a retrospective observational study. Lancet Neurol. 2012;11(9):784-91.
38. Rathore C, Sarma SP, Radhakrishnan K. Prognostic importance of serial postoperative EEGs after anterior temporal lobectomy. Neurology. 2011;76(22):1925-31.
39. Lamberink HJ, Boshuisen K, Otte WM, Geleijns K, Braun KPJ; TimeToStop Study Group. Individualized prediction of seizure relapse and outcomes following antiepileptic drug withdrawal after pediatric epilepsy surgery. Epilepsia. 2018;59(3):e28-33.
40. Rathore C, Radhakrishnan K, Jeyaraj MK, Wattamwar PR, Baheti N, Sarma SP. Early versus late antiepileptic drug withdrawal following temporal lobectomy. Seizure. 2020;75:23-7.
41. Brodie MJ, Kwan P. Epilepsy in elderly people. BMJ. 2005;331(7528):1317-22.
42. Panayiotopoulos CP, Obeid T, Tahan AR. Juvenile myoclonic epilepsy: a 5-year prospective study. Epilepsia. 1994;35(2):285-96.
43. Pavlović M, Jović N, Pekmezović T. Antiepileptic drugs withdrawal in patients with idiopathic generalized epilepsy. Seizure. 2011;20(7):520-5.
44. Senf P, Schmitz B, Holtkamp M, Janz D. Prognosis of juvenile myoclonic epilepsy 45 years after onset: seizure outcome and predictors. Neurology. 2013;81(24):2128-33.
45. Geithner J, Schneider F, Wang Z, Berneiser J, Herzer R, Kessler C, et al. Predictors for long-term seizure outcome in juvenile myoclonic epilepsy: 25–63 years of follow-up. Epilepsia. 2012;53(8):1379-86.
46. Gupta M, Agarwal P, Khwaja GA, Chowdhury D, Sharma B, Bansal J, et al. Randomized prospective study of outcome of short term antiepileptic treatment in small single enhancing CT lesion in brain. Neurol India. 2002;50(2):145-7.
47. Thussu A, Arora A, Prabhakar S, Lal V, Sawhney IM. Acute symptomatic seizures due to single CT lesions: how long to treat with antiepileptic drugs? Neurol India. 2002;50(2):141-4.
48. Rajshekhar V, Jeyaseelan L. Seizure outcome in patients with a solitary cerebral cysticercus granuloma. Neurology. 2004;62(12):2236-40.
49. Hesdorffer DC, Benn EK, Cascino GD, Hauser WA. Is a first acute symptomatic seizure epilepsy? Mortality and risk for recurrent seizure. Epilepsia. 2009;50(5):1102-8.
50. Hesdorffer DC, Logroscino G, Cascino G, Annegers JF, Hauser WA. Risk of unprovoked seizure after acute symptomatic seizure: effect of status epilepticus. Ann Neurol. 1998;44(6):908-12.
51. Gunawardane N, Fields M. Acute symptomatic seizures and provoked seizures: to Treat or Not to Treat? Curr Treat Options Neurol. 2018;20(10):41.
52. Sawhney IM, McLauchlan DJ, Powell HWR. Management of acute symptomatic seizures: outline of current practice. JNNP. 2012;83 (Suppl 2):A4.

CHAPTER 7

Management of Surgically Remediable Epilepsy

S Sidharth, P Sarat Chandra, Manjari Tripathi

ABSTRACT

This chapter provides a comprehensive overview of the management of surgically remediable epilepsy, focusing on drug-resistant epilepsy (DRE). It details the presurgical evaluation process, including patient history, video electroencephalography (EEG) monitoring, neuroimaging, and neuropsychological testing. The chapter also discusses the importance of identifying the epileptogenic zone (EZ) and presents various diagnostic tools and multidisciplinary approaches used to pinpoint this zone. Additionally, it outlines the different types of epilepsy surgeries and neuromodulation techniques, and highlights the significance of diet therapy in managing DRE, with emphasizing the need for tailored surgical interventions and the importance of comprehensive evaluation in improving patient outcomes.

Keywords: Drug resistant epilepsy, Epileptogenic zone, Level 1, Level 2, Stereo-electroencephalography, Resective surgery, Neuromodulation.

■ INTRODUCTION

Epilepsy surgery is an option for patients with drug-resistant epilepsy (DRE), where seizures remain uncontrolled despite optimal medical therapy. Approximately one-third of people with epilepsy have DRE, significantly impacting their quality of life (QOL). The presurgical evaluation aims to identify the epileptogenic zone (EZ) to achieve seizure freedom without causing unacceptable functional deficits. This chapter discusses the comprehensive approach to managing surgically remediable epilepsy, including diagnostic tools, surgical techniques, and alternative treatments such as neuromodulation and diet therapy.

■ WHAT IS DRUG-RESISTANT EPILEPSY?

Drug-resistant epilepsy, also known as intractable or pharmacoresistant epilepsy, is defined as the failure to achieve seizure control despite the use of two or more appropriately chosen and adequately dosed antiseizure medications (ASMs).[1]

Approximately one-third of people with epilepsy have DRE which impacts their QOL. The underlying causes of DRE can include structural brain abnormalities, genetic factors, and other unknown reasons. Advanced treatment for DRE like surgical interventions, become necessary to achieve better seizure control.[2]

WHAT IS PSEUDOREFRACTORY EPILEPSY?

Pseudorefractory epilepsy[3] occurs when seizures are resistant to treatment due to factors other than true pharmacoresistance. These factors can include incorrect diagnosis, improper drug choice, poor medication adherence, or incorrect dosages. Addressing these issues can sometimes make seemingly DRE treatable. For example, an incorrect diagnosis of epilepsy might be made when a patient actually has a different condition that mimics seizures, like psychogenic nonepileptic seizures (PNES).

PRESURGICAL EVALUATION

Presurgical evaluation is a comprehensive process designed to determine if a person with DRE is a candidate for surgery. This evaluation aims to localize the EZ and ensure that its removal will not cause unacceptable functional deficits.

The objective of epilepsy surgery is the complete resection or disconnection of the EZ, the area of the cortex necessary for the generation of habitual seizures and the smallest amount of tissue that can be removed to achieve a seizure-free outcome.

The EZ is a theoretical construct and there is no established marker that definitively determines its location and extent. The EZ can only be estimated through a variety of diagnostic tests that point out different cortical zones that are considered more or less precise indicators of the EZ **(Fig. 1)**:[4]

- *Seizure-onset zone (SOZ):* The area where the clinical seizures originate on ictal recordings.
- *Irritative zone:* The area of the cortex that generates interictal epileptiform discharges (IEDs) in the electroencephalography (EEG) or magnetoencephalography (MEG).
- *Epileptogenic lesion:* A structural brain abnormality that is causally related to epilepsy.
- *Functional deficit zone*: The area of the cortex that is functionally abnormal during the interictal period, as indicated by neurological examination, neuropsychological testing, and functional imaging.

The process involves multiple diagnostic tools and a multidisciplinary approach, including:
- *Patient history and clinical examination:* Detailed documentation of seizure types

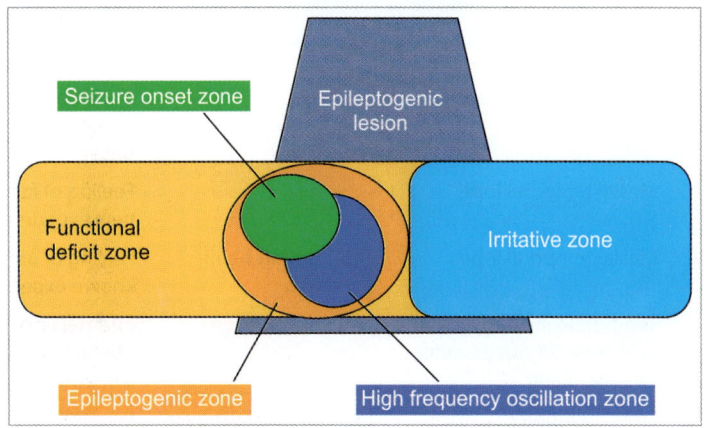

FIG. 1: Different zones with respect to the epileptogenic lesion.

and semiology, frequency, triggers, and previous treatments. This helps in clinical localization and hypothesis formulation.
- *Video-EEG (VEEG) monitoring:* Long-term monitoring captures seizures to correlate clinical and electrical findings.

The International League Against Epilepsy (ILAE) provides specific guidelines for the minimum recommended duration of VEEG monitoring and the number of events needed for each semiology.[5]
- *Minimum duration of VEEG monitoring:* The ILAE recommends a minimum duration of 72 hours (3 days) for VEEG monitoring.[5] This time frame allows for the capture of a sufficient number of habitual seizures and IEDs, which are crucial for accurate diagnosis and treatment planning.
- *Number of events required:* The ILAE suggests that at least 3–5 events of each semiology are necessary to ensure accurate localization and differentiation of seizure types. Capturing multiple events helps to confirm the consistency of the seizure onset zone and the associated semiology.
- *Tapering of ASMs during VEEG:*
  - *Daily seizure:* Observe for 1 day, if no seizure, taper by 10–25% of total dose.
  - *Weekly seizure:* Taper by 25–30% of dose.
  - *Monthly seizure:* Taper by 50% of total dose.
- *Neuroimaging:* High-resolution magnetic resonance imaging (MRI) with epilepsy-specific protocols to identify structural abnormalities.
- *Neuropsychological testing:* To evaluate cognitive functions and help predict the impact of surgery.
- *Multidisciplinary team review:* Involves neurologists, neurosurgeons, neuropsychologists, and radiologists.

■ HYPOTHESIS FORMULATION

Hypothesis forming integrates multiple data points to pinpoint the EZ. This involves:
- *Clinical symptoms*: Detailed descriptions of seizures, including onset, duration, and progression. Detailed semiology[6] is given in **Tables 1 and 2** further.

TABLE 1: Semiology description with localization, lateralization.[6]

Semiology feature	Localization	Lateralization	Description
Aura	Temporal lobe	–	Sensory, autonomic, or psychic phenomena experienced before a seizure onset
Déjà vu	Mesial temporal lobe	–	Feeling of familiarity with a new experience
Jamais vu	Mesial temporal lobe	Typically left hemisphere	Feeling of unfamiliarity with a known experience
Fear	Temporal lobe (amygdala, orbitofrontal cortex, anterior cingulate)	Either (right > left)	Intense, unpleasant emotion due to belief that someone or something is dangerous
Eye blinking	Frontotemporal	Ipsilateral hemisphere if unilateral blink	Repetitive tonic contraction of eyelids

Continued

Continued

Semiology feature	Localization	Lateralization	Description
Epigastric rising sensation	Mesial temporal lobe	–	Rising sensation in the abdomen often preceding a seizure
Olfactory hallucinations	Mesial temporal lobe, frontal lobe, insula	–	Perception of smells that are not present (e.g., burnt rubber)
Auditory hallucinations	Temporal lobe (posterior superior temporal neocortex)	–	Hearing sounds or voices that are not present
Gestural automatisms	Temporal	Ipsilateral	Repetitive, purposeless movements like hand-rubbing
Aphasia	Dominant hemisphere	Broca's, Wernicke's, Basal temporal language area	Inability to comprehend or formulate language
Hypermotor seizures	Frontal lobe	Often lateralized	Violent, vigorous movements such as thrashing or kicking
Tonic posturing	Supplementary motor area	Typically contralateral	Sustained muscle contractions resulting in rigid posturing
Figure of four posture	Premotor and motor cortex	Contralateral to extended arm	Extension of one arm, flexion of other arm
Clonic movements	Primary motor cortex	Typically contralateral	Rhythmic jerking movements
Versive movements	Frontal lobe	Contralateral to head turn	Forced, sustained turning of the head and eyes to one side
Ictal speech arrest	Dominant hemisphere (frontal)	Typically lateralized	Sudden inability to speak during a seizure
Sensory disturbances	Parietal lobe	Contralateral to sensory changes	Numbness, tingling, or other altered sensations
Visual hallucinations	Occipital lobe	Contralateral visual cortex	Seeing lights, shapes, or people that are not present
Gelastic seizures	Hypothalamus	–	Episodes of inappropriate laughter
Dacrystic seizures	Temporal lobe	–	Episodes of crying or sobbing without an apparent emotional trigger
Focal impaired awareness seizures	Temporal or frontal lobe	• Complete impairment: Dominant lobe • Partial impairment: Nondominant lobe	Impairment of consciousness with or without motor manifestations
Generalized tonic-clonic seizures	Multiple regions	Bilateral	Loss of consciousness with initial tonic stiffening followed by clonic jerking

TABLE 2: Postictal phenomenon and their localization.

Postictal phenomenon	Localization
Postictal headache	Ipsilateral (in context to temporal lobe epilepsy)
Postictal aphasia	Dominant hemisphere
Postictal nose wiping	Ipsilateral (in context to temporal lobe epilepsy)
Postictal paresis (Todd's)	Contralateral

- *Home videos:* Family members are counseled to make home video recordings of seizure events providing valuable information about seizure semiology. Most of the time, the bystander who has witnessed the seizure may not accurately remember the sequence of semiology, and thus making home videos and bringing it to the clinic may supplement the hypothesis formulation for localization.
- *Interictal EEG:* EEG recordings between seizures showing IEDs to localize the irritative zone.
- *Ictal EEG:* EEG during seizures to localize the seizure onset zone.
- *Epilepsy protocol MRI:* High-resolution imaging to identify structural abnormalities.

WHICH PATIENTS CAN BE TAKEN UP FOR SURGERY BY VIDEO ELECTROENCEPHALOGRAPHY AND MAGNETIC RESONANCE IMAGING?

Patients considered for epilepsy surgery typically meet the following criteria:[7]
- Clear identification of the EZ through VEEG and MRI.
- Localization of the seizure focus to a single, resectable area of the brain with concordance demonstrated.

TABLE 3: Misconceptions about epilepsy surgery versus fact.[8]

Misconception	Fact
All ASM need to be tried	Chance of seizure remission is <10% after two drugs have failed
Bilateral EEG spikes are contraindication to surgery	Unilateral seizure onset commonly have bilateral interictal spikes
Normal MRI as contraindication	Other advanced techniques often detect a single epileptogenic zone with normal MRI
Multiple or diffuse lesions on MRI as contraindication	Epileptogenic zone may involve one or a part of the lesion
Surgery not possible if eloquent cortex is involved	Risk-benefit ratio can be individualized
IQ <70 is a contraindication to surgery	May benefit from remission or reduction in seizures

(ASM: antiseizure medicine; EEG: electroencephalography; IQ: intelligence quotient; MRI: magnetic resonance imaging)

- No evidence of diffuse or multifocal epilepsy, which would make surgical intervention less likely to be successful.
- Favorable risk-benefit ratio, ensuring that resection will not lead to significant neurological deficits.

Table 3 shows misconceptions about epilepsy surgery versus fact.[8]

NEUROIMAGING IN EPILEPSY

Overview

The Harmonized Neuroimaging of Epilepsy Structural Sequences (HARNESS)[9] protocol is a consensus-based recommendation developed by ILAE to standardize the use of structural MRI in the diagnosis and management of epilepsy. It is designed to optimize lesion detection and improve clinical decision-making, particularly in patients with DRE.

HARNESS protocol includes:
- *3D T1-weighted MRI:* Includes magnetization-prepared rapid gradient-echo (MP-RAGE) or equivalent sequences. It is optimal for evaluating brain anatomy and morphology.
- *3D fluid-attenuated inversion recovery (FLAIR):* It is best suited for detecting signal anomalies such as gliosis and hyperintensities. Nulls cerebrospinal fluid (CSF) signal to enhance visibility of cortical lesions.
- *2D coronal T2-weighted MRI:* It includes turbo spin echo sequence for detailed hippocampal assessment. Images are acquired perpendicular to the hippocampus's long axis with submillimetric voxel resolution.

TABLE 4: Magnetic resonance imaging sequences with the conditions.

T1	High resolution anatomical details to detect cortical dysplasia, tumors, and atrophy
T2	Hippocampal sclerosis, tumors, and edema
T2 FLAIR	Cortical dysplasia, gliosis
T2 GRE	*Detects hemosiderin deposits: Cavernous malformations*
DWI	Acute ischemic lesions and cytotoxic edema
Magnetic resonance spectroscopy	Biochemical change like N-acetyl aspartate levels indicating neuronal loss

(DWI: diffusion-weighted imaging; FLAIR: fluid attenuated inversion recovery; GRE: gradient-echo)

Key Points

- *Applicability:* HARNESS protocol is suitable for both adults and children. It can be *performed on 1.5T and 3T MRI scanners, though optimized for 3T.*
- *Time-efficient:* Each sequence lasts 7–10 minutes. Total acquisition time is under 30 minutes.
- *High-resolution imaging:* Utilizes high-contrast, 3D sequences with isotropic voxels ($1 \times 1 \times 1$ mm³). It provides complete brain coverage without the need for operator-dependent slice angulations. Images can be reformatted in any plane without loss of resolution.
- *Improved detection:* It reduces partial volume effects, enhancing signal-to-noise ratio and tissue contrast.
- *Repeat imaging:* ILAE recommends repeating MRI using the HARNESS protocol if previous investigations were unremarkable or suboptimal.

Note: HARNESS MRI protocol should be complemented with:
- *T1 MRI with gadolinium:* When a tumor, vascular malformation, or infectious process is suspected to look for contrast enhancement.
- *Susceptibility-weighted imaging and T2 contrasts:* Sensitive to venous blood, *hemorrhage, iron deposits, and calcifications.*

Table 4 showing MRI sequences with the conditions identified.

■ WHEN TO REFER TO A LEVEL 2 CENTER

Referral to a specialized epilepsy center (level 2) is recommended when noninvasive evaluations are inconclusive or advanced diagnostic tools are required. The referral should be done if the presurgical evaluations reveal multiple seizure foci, discordance between VEEG and the structural lesion, when the resection involves close to the eloquent cortex.

Table 5 shows recommendation of level 1 and level 2 epilepsy center for surgical management of epilepsy.[10]

Presurgical Evaluation Tool for Refractory Epilepsy

The presurgical evaluation tool for refractory epilepsy (PETRE) tool is designed to predict

TABLE 5: Level 1 and level 2 epilepsy center for surgical management of epilepsy.

Capability	Level 1 center	Level 2 center
Electrodiagnostic	>24 hours VEEG and EEG with surface/sphenoidal recording	All level 1 capabilities plus: 24-hour video/EEG with invasive monitoring, evoked potential recording, electrocorticography
Epilepsy surgery	Emergency or elective neurosurgery, mesial temporal sclerosis, referral agreements with level 2 centers	• All level 1 capabilities plus: Clinical experience of >25 cases per year • Invasive monitoring: SEEG
Imaging	MRI with fMRI for language and memory	Both standard and special investigations (PET, SPECT, and MEG)
Pharmacological expertise	Quality-assured antiepileptic drug levels, 24-hour antiepileptic drug level service	Same as level 1
Neuropsychological/psychosocial services	Available	Same as level 1
Rehabilitation	Inpatient and outpatient services	Same as level 1
Mandatory expertise	Neurosurgery, neurology, internal medicine, pediatrics, and general surgery	All level 1 experts plus: Neuroradiologist, nuclear medicine specialist, psychiatrist

(fMRI: functional magnetic resonance imaging; MEG: magnetoencephalography; PET: positron emission tomography; SPECT: single-photon-emission computed tomography; SEEG: stereoelectroencephalography; VEEG: video-electroencephalography)

surgical candidacy in DRE patients by evaluating variables such as seizure severity, MRI and EEG findings, seizure duration, number of antiepileptic drugs (AEDs) tried, and their side effects. It helps streamline the evaluation process, particularly in resource-limited settings, ensuring timely identification of patients who would benefit from epilepsy surgery. A prospective study[11] aimed to expedite epilepsy surgery evaluations by developing the PETRE to identify surgical candidates among 501 DRE at a tertiary care center in India. Key predictors of surgical candidacy included disabling seizures, lesional MRI, higher number of AEDs, and longer seizure duration. PETRE, validated in 40 DRE individuals proved valuable in optimizing epilepsy monitoring unit (EMU) resource use and improving patient management in resource-limited settings, offering a quick guide to identify potential surgical candidates.

Phase 1 Investigations[7]

- High-resolution MRI
- Video scalp EEG
- *Detailed neuropsychological assessment:* To evaluate cognitive functions and predict the impact of surgery on these functions. Standardized tests to assess memory, language, attention, and executive functions. Provides information on potential postoperative deficits and aids in surgical decision-making.

Additional Phase 1 Investigations If Results are Ambiguous[7]

- *Interictal high-resolution EEG (HD-EEG):* Enhanced spatial resolution to better localize the irritative zone.
- *Interictal MEG:* Localizes magnetic fields generated by neuronal activity.
- *Interictal EEG-functional MRI (EEG-fMRI):* Maps hemodynamic changes related to epileptic activity.

- *Interictal positron emission tomography (PET) [18F-fluorodeoxyglucose (FDG)] or other tracers:* Identifies functional deficit zones through hypometabolism.
- *Ictal single-photon-emission computed tomography (SPECT):* Measures changes in regional cerebral blood flow during seizures to localize the ictal onset zone.

Ictal and Interictal Electroencephalography

The EEG, both ictal (during seizures) and interictal (between seizures), is fundamental in localizing seizure onset and identifying EZs.

Indications:[12] Interictal EEG helps in identifying potential epileptic regions, while ictal EEG provides direct evidence of seizure onset.

Recommendations: Continuous VEEG monitoring is recommended for comprehensive evaluation, especially in patients with refractory epilepsy.

Positron Emission Tomography

The PET imaging is typically performed interictally to identify hypometabolism as a marker of cortical dysfunction.

Indications:[12] PET is useful when MRI does not identify a lesion that is concordant with clinical and EEG data. It helps in hemispheric lateralization and general lobar localization, especially in cases with discordant scalp EEG or normal MRI.

Recommendations: PET imaging, specifically with 18F-FDG, is recommended for better anatomical and functional information. It has a sensitivity of up to 90% in temporal lobe epilepsy and about 50% in extratemporal lobe epilepsy.

Single Photon Emission Computed Tomography

The SPECT imaging uses technetium-99m-labeled ligands to measure regional cerebral blood flow. It is performed both interictally and ictally to visualize areas of hyperperfusion associated with seizure onset.

Indications:[12] Ictal SPECT is crucial for identifying the seizure onset zone, while interictal SPECT aids in detecting hyperperfusion due to seizure propagation.

SISCOM: Use of ictal and interictal SPECT with coregistration to MRI (SISCOM) for improved sensitivity.

Ictal SPECT had a 70% sensitivity compared to 78% with interictal 18F- FDG PET. When ictal and interictal SPECT are normalized and subtracted, the sensitivity of SPECT has reached 87%.[13]

Chandra et al.[14] evaluated the role of interconcordance between FDG-PET and ictal-SPECT in predicting long-term outcomes after epilepsy surgery in 123 individuals with DRE. Results showed that for extra-temporal epilepsies, concordance between FDG-PET, Ictal-SPECT, MRI, and VEEG significantly predicted better 5-year outcomes (62% seizure-free) compared to other situations ($p < 0.01$). In temporal epilepsies, MRI and VEEG were the most crucial prognostic factors, with concordance correlating to improved outcomes in both temporal (70% vs. 25%) and extra-temporal (62% vs. 33%) cases ($p < 0.05$).

Magnetoencephalography

The MEG measures the magnetic fields generated by neuronal activity, providing high spatial and temporal resolution of cortical sources.

Indications:[12] MEG is useful for localizing interictal epileptic activity and is particularly beneficial when scalp EEG is inconclusive or when deeper cortical sources need to be evaluated.

Recommendations: MEG should be used to complement other imaging modalities for precise localization of epileptic zones, especially when planning for intracranial EEG (IEEG).

The study by Kaur et al.[15] investigated the diagnostic performance and utility of MEG and SPECT in presurgical evaluation of DRE. The study included a sample size of 102 DRE, with common etiologies being focal cortical dysplasia (FCD) in 44 patients, mesial temporal sclerosis (MTS) in 11 patients, and ganglioglioma/dysembryoplastic neuroepithelial tumor (DNET) in six patients. This study indicated that SPECT had a marginally better diagnostic yield compared to MEG, with a higher sensitivity (83.3% vs. 79.5%) and accuracy (78.57% vs. 74.26%). However, MEG was more accessible and easier to obtain, providing significant value in localizing the EZ, especially in cases where SPECT could not be performed.

Phase 2 Investigations[7]

- *Intracranial EEG:* To achieve precise localization of the EZ when noninvasive methods are insufficient. It provides high spatial resolution for identifying the seizure onset zone.
- *Extraoperative IEEG (CEEG):* Subdural grids or strips placed through open craniotomy.
- *Stereoelectroencephalography (SEEG):* Depth electrodes placed stereotactically for recording.
- *Hybrid extraoperative EEG (HEEG):* Combination of CEEG and SEEG.
- *Intraoperative electrocorticography (ECoG):* To map and monitor electrical activity intraoperatively by subdural, depth, or wick electrodes placed during surgery. This helps the surgeon to guide resection while minimizing damage to essential brain areas.
- *Functional MRI:* Maps functional areas and predicts postoperative cognitive outcomes. Mainly used for localization of eloquent cortex and prediction of language and memory outcomes. fMRI has replaced the Wada test in many centers for language lateralization.
- *Magnetic source imaging (MSI):* Combines MEG and MRI for precise localization of EZs. Useful for planning IEEG placement and surgical resection.

A prospective observational study[16] with 102 people with epilepsy underwent epilepsy surgery. A total of 76% of the patients underwent surgical resection in sublobes concordant with MSI localization, and the diagnostic odds ratio for good (Engel I) outcome in these patients was 2.3 (95% confidence interval 0.68, 7.86; $p = 0.183$) after long-term follow-up of 36 months.

Stereoelectroencephalography

The SEEG involves the placement of depth electrodes to record electrical activity directly from the brain tissue, providing high-spatial resolution.

Indications:[12] SEEG is indicated for patients with complex focal epilepsy where noninvasive methods fail to localize the seizure onset zone. It is especially useful in cases with multiple or deep-seated foci.

Recommendations: SEEG should be employed when hypothesis-driven localization is necessary, particularly in cases where precise mapping of epileptic zones is critical for surgical planning **Flowchart 1**.[10]

■ CLINICAL ALGORITHM FOR PRESURGICAL EVALUATION (FLOWCHART 2)

Refer to **Flowchart 2**.[10]

■ CONCEPT OF ROBOTIC THERMOCOAGULATIVE HEMISPHEROTOMY

A novel "bloodless" minimally invasive robotic thermocoagulative hemispherotomy

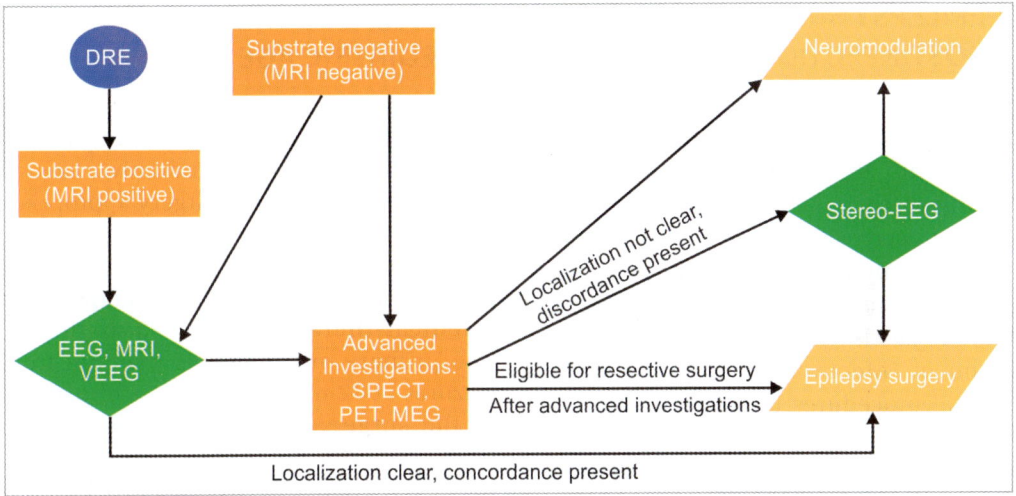

FLOWCHART 1: Flowchart for surgical management in DRE.
(DRE: drug-resistant epilepsy; EEG: electroencephalography; fMRI: functional magnetic resonance imaging; MEG: magnetoencephalography; MRI: magnetic resonance imaging; PET: positron emission tomography; SEEG: stereoelectroencephalography; SPECT: single-photon-emission computed tomography)

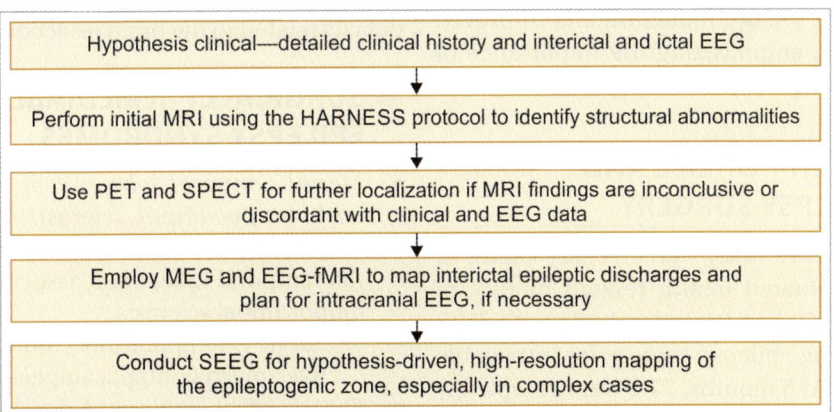

FLOWCHART 2: Algorithm for presurgical evaluation.
(EEG: electroencephalography; fMRI: functional magnetic resonance imaging; HARNESS: Harmonized Neuroimaging of Epilepsy Structural Sequences; MEG: magnetoencephalography; MRI: magnetic resonance imaging; PET: positron emission tomography; SEEG: stereoelectroencephalography; SPECT: single-photon-emission computed tomography)

(ROTCH),[17] first described by Prof Sarat Chandra, involves using a robotic system to plan five sets of trajectories for anterior, middle, and posterior disconnections, corpus callosotomy, and temporal stem and amygdala disconnection. Six patients with various pathologies underwent the procedure, with a mean follow-up of 13.5 months. The outcomes were promising, with 83% achieving class 1 outcomes on the ILAE Outcome Scale and estimated blood loss under 5 mL for all patients. Complications were minimal, including one repeat surgery and one resolving temporal hematoma. ROTCH appears to be a safe and effective procedure with very low morbidity.

EPILEPSY SURGERY IN POSTINFECTIOUS ETIOLOGY

The DRE due to postinfectious etiologies in 28 patients was evaluated in an observational study[18] with etiologies being postpyogenic meningitic/encephalitic sequelae (8 cases), neurocysticercosis (6 cases), tuberculomas/post-tuberculous (4 cases), postpyogenic abscess (4 cases), post-traumatic abscess-related gliosis (2 cases), and gliosis of unknown infectious etiology (4 cases). Surgical procedures included mesial temporal lobectomy, lateral temporal, frontal, and parietal resections, and hemispherotomy. At an average follow-up of 14.2 months, 81% of patients achieved a good outcome (Engel class I or II), with 60% reaching Engel class I. The study concludes that surgery for DRE due to postinfectious etiologies can lead to significant seizure reduction and improved outcomes, emphasizing the importance of early identification and intervention.

QUALITY OF LIFE AND EPILEPSY SURGERY

A prospective study[19] at a tertiary center in India evaluated health-related quality of life (HRQOL) in 36 individuals with DRE undergoing epilepsy surgery for intractable seizures. At 6 months, 77% were completely seizure-free. Significant HRQOL improvements were observed in all domains for individuals with good seizure outcomes (Engel 1 and 2). Even individuals with poor seizure outcomes (Engel 3 and 4) showed significant improvements in seizure worry, overall QOL, emotional wellbeing, energy fatigue, and social functioning. Complete seizure freedom was strongly associated with greater HRQOL improvements and even in individuals not achieving good seizure outcome had improvement in HRQOL parameters mentioned earlier by QOLIE-31.

EPILEPSY SURGERY IN PEDIATRIC AGE GROUPS

A single center randomized trial by Dwivedi et al.[20] involving 116 DRE aged 18 or younger. The participants were randomly assigned to either undergo brain surgery appropriate to the underlying cause of epilepsy along with medical therapy (surgery group, 57 patients) or receive medical therapy alone (medical-therapy group, 59 patients). The primary outcome was freedom from seizures at 12 months with 77% of patients in the surgery group achieving freedom from seizures compared to 7% in the medical-therapy group ($p < 0.001$). The study concluded that epilepsy surgery in children and adolescents with DRE resulted in higher rates of seizure freedom and better behavioral and QOL outcomes compared to medical therapy alone, despite anticipated neurologic deficits related to the brain resection.

SURGICALLY REMEDIABLE EPILEPSY SYNDROMES

- *Mesial temporal lobe epilepsy (MTLE) with hippocampal sclerosis:* Seizures originating from the mesial structures of the temporal lobe, often associated with hippocampal sclerosis.
    - Surgery: Temporal lobectomy or selective amygdalohippocampectomy.[21]
- *Focal cortical dysplasia:* A developmental anomaly where the brain cortex is malformed, leading to focal seizures.
    - Surgery: Resection of the dysplastic brain tissue.
- *Tuberous sclerosis complex (TSC):* A genetic disorder causing benign tumors to form in various organs, including the brain, leading to epilepsy. Seizures vary widely, including infantile spasms, focal seizures, and generalized seizures.
    - Surgery: Resection of tubers or focal areas causing seizures, and in some cases, vagus nerve stimulation (VNS) or responsive neurostimulation (RNS).[22]

- *Rasmussen's encephalitis:* A rare, chronic inflammatory disease affecting one hemisphere of the brain, leading to progressive neurological decline and intractable seizures. It usually presents with focal seizures, hemiparesis, and cognitive decline.
  - *Surgery:* Functional hemispherectomy or hemispherotomy.[17]
- *Sturge–Weber syndrome:* A neurocutaneous disorder with vascular malformations in the brain leading to seizures. It presents with focal seizures, often associated with a facial port-wine stain and glaucoma.
  - *Surgery:* Resection of the affected brain area or functional hemispherotomy.[17]
- *Hypothalamic hamartoma:* A benign tumor in the hypothalamus causing gelastic (laughing) seizures and other seizure types. It presents with gelastic seizures, cognitive and behavioral issues.
  - *Surgery:* Surgical resection/disconnection, radiofrequency ablation, or laser interstitial thermal therapy (LITT).[17]
- *Periventricular nodular heterotopia:* A condition where neurons fail to migrate properly during brain development, leading to nodules along the ventricular walls.
  - *Surgery:* Resection of the EZ.[17]
- *Polymicrogyria:* A malformation characterized by an excessive number of small, abnormal gyri in the brain. Varied seizure types ranging from focal seizures to focal to bilateral tonic clonic seizures.
  - *Surgery:* Resection of affected areas if they can be localized as the seizure focus.[17]
- *Epilepsy associated with low-grade brain tumors:* Tumors such as gangliogliomas or DNETs can cause epilepsy.
  - *Surgery:* Tumor resection can often control seizures.[17]
- *Hemimegalencephaly:* A rare congenital condition where one cerebral hemisphere is abnormally larger than the other, often leading to intractable seizures. Severe seizures, developmental delays, and hemiparesis.
  - *Surgery:* Functional hemispherectomy or hemispherotomy.[17]
- *Lennox–Gastaut syndrome (LGS):* A severe epilepsy syndrome that begins in childhood and is characterized by multiple types of seizures and intellectual disability. Genetic mutations may be involved. Seizure types include atypical absence seizures, tonic seizures, and atonic seizures.
  - *Surgery:* Corpus callosotomy, posterior disconnection, and VNS.[23]

NEUROMODULATION IN TREATMENT OF DRUG-RESISTANT EPILEPSY

Neuromodulation refers to electrical stimulation of the nervous system to modulate specific functions such as movement disorders, pain, and epilepsy. For patients with DRE, where resection or disconnection surgery is not possible, neuromodulation provides an alternative treatment option.

Types of Neuromodulation (Table 6)[30]

- *Vagal nerve stimulation:* VNS stimulates the vagus nerve, which is believed to reduce seizure activity by decreasing hyperemia and desynchronizing seizure network activity. It also affects neurotransmitter release, increasing Gamma-aminobutyric acid (GABA) and decreasing glutamate levels. VNS was approved by the Food and Drug administration (FDA) in 1997 for patients older than 12 years, and in 2017 for children over 4 years with partial seizures.[24] A generator implanted in the chest wall stimulates the vagus nerve intermittently. It provides significant seizure reduction but rarely

TABLE 6: Summary of the neuromodulation techniques.[30]

Device type	Mechanism	Application	Efficacy	Adverse effects
VNS	Vagus nerve stimulation	Partial seizures in adults and children	Significant seizure reduction, rarely seizure-free	Implant site pain, infection
DBS	Deep brain stimulation	Temporal lobe epilepsy, generalized seizures	Significant seizure reduction, improved quality of life (QOL)	Battery changes, target mismatch
RNS	Responsive neurostimulation	Refractory focal epilepsy	Sustained seizure reduction	Paresthesia, implant site pain
TNS	Trigeminal nerve stimulation	Drug-resistant epilepsy	Promising seizure reduction	Minimal adverse effects
rTMS	Repetitive transcranial magnetic stimulation	Cortical dysplasia	Significant seizure reduction	Headache
tDCS	Transcranial direct current stimulation	Mesial temporal sclerosis	High responder rates	Minimal adverse effects

complete seizure freedom and is widely available and used globally. This is to be done after ruling out all possibility of resective surgery by all possible investigations (VEEG, MRI, SISCOM, PET, MEG, and SEEG), wherever applicable. In Indian setting, it is often done for bilateral hypoxic ischemic damage where there are bilateral onset seizures or LGS secondary to diffuse etiologies.

- *Deep brain stimulation (DBS):* Electrodes are implanted into deeper brain targets to disrupt seizure activity through high-frequency stimulation. It affects ion channels and neurotransmitter levels, altering network excitability. It was approved in Europe in 2010 and by the US FDA in 2018 for DRE.[25] Targets include the anterior nucleus of the thalamus (ANT) and centromedian nucleus of thalamus (CMNT). It reduces seizures significantly, especially in temporal lobe epilepsy, with improvements in QOL. However, it requires frequent battery changes and is more expensive than VNS.
- *Responsive neurostimulation:* RNS includes electrodes that record electrocorticogram data and deliver electrical stimuli to the seizure focus upon detecting epileptiform activity. It operates in a closed-loop system without human intervention. It was approved by the US FDA in 2013 for adults with refractory focal epilepsy with up to two identified seizure foci.[26] It provides significant seizure reduction and valuable electrophysiological data for research. Long-term follow-up studies show sustained efficacy. This is not available in India as yet.
- *Trigeminal nerve stimulation (TNS):* Noninvasive bilateral stimulation of the supraorbital nerves. High-frequency stimulation shows better efficacy in reducing seizures. It is an economical and easily applicable technique with promising results in reducing seizure frequency with ongoing research for long-term efficacy.[27]
- *Repetitive transcranial magnetic stimulation (rTMS):* It uses magnetic fields to induce electrical currents that affect neuronal activity. Repetition leads to longer-lasting effects. It is effective in reducing seizures, especially in cortical dysplasia.[28]
- *Transcranial direct current stimulation (tDCS):* Portable, noninvasive technique

that uses weak direct current to influence cortical excitability. It is effective in reducing seizures in MTS. It showed promising results with high responder rates but requires further long-term studies.[29]

DIET THERAPY IN DRUG-RESISTANT EPILEPSY

Diet therapy has become an important alternative treatment for patients with DRE. These dietary treatments have shown effectiveness in reducing seizure frequency and improving the QOL in patients who do not respond to traditional AEDs.

Types of Diet Therapy

- *Ketogenic diet (KD):* A high-fat, low-carbohydrate, and adequate-protein diet that induces a state of ketosis, where the body uses fat instead of carbohydrates for energy.[30]
  - *Mechanism:* Ketosis is believed to stabilize neuronal activity and reduce seizure frequency.
  - *Efficacy:* The classic KD is highly effective, particularly in children, with many experiencing a 50% or greater reduction in seizures. Some patients achieve complete seizure freedom. It is primarily used in children with DRE but can be effective in adults.
- *Modified Atkins diet (MAD):* A less restrictive version of the KD that allows more protein and fewer restrictions on fluid and calorie intake.
  - *Mechanism:* Similar to the KD, it induces ketosis but is easier to follow.
  - *Efficacy:* Effective in reducing seizures, with a significant number of patients experiencing a 50% or greater reduction in seizure frequency. It is suitable for adolescents and adults with DRE due to its flexibility and ease of implementation.[31,32]
- *Low glycemic index treatment (LGIT):* Focuses on controlling blood glucose levels by using foods with a low glycemic index, which have a slower impact on blood sugar. An option for patients who may have difficulty adhering to the strict KD or MAD.
- *Medium chain triglyceride (MCT) diet:* Utilizes MCTs to produce ketones, allowing for a higher carbohydrate intake compared to the classic KD. Suitable for patients who struggle with the strictness of the classic KD.

Implementation and Monitoring

- *Initial assessment:* Before starting diet therapy, a comprehensive assessment by a multidisciplinary team is essential to determine the appropriate dietary regimen.
- *Monitoring:* Regular follow-up is necessary to monitor nutritional status, growth (in children), and potential side effects such as gastrointestinal disturbances, hyperlipidemia, and kidney stones.
- *Adjustments:* Diets may need to be adjusted based on individual tolerance, efficacy in seizure control, and patient preference.

CONCLUSION

Presurgical evaluation of drug resistant epilepsy should be done timely with level 1 and level 2 investigations. Use of advanced investigations in multiple epileptogenic zones, discordant VEEG and MRI, MRI negative epilepsy should be done for deciding the surgical approach. Epilepsy surgery with resection, lesionectomy, stereo-electroencephalogram guided ablation, neuromodulation techniques are available. Diet therapy may act as an adjuvant therapy where surgery may not be possible.

REFERENCES

1. Kwan P, Arzimanoglou A, Berg AT, Brodie MJ, Allen Hauser W, Mathern G, et al. Definition of drug resistant epilepsy: consensus proposal by the ad hoc Task Force of the ILAE Commission on Therapeutic Strategies. Epilepsia. 2010;51(6): 1069-77.
2. Engel J. Surgical treatment for epilepsy: Too little, Too late? JAMA. 2008;300(21):2548-50.
3. Lazarus JP, Bhatia M, Shukla G, Padma MV, Tripathi M, Srivastava AK, et al. A study of non-epileptic seizures in an Indian population. Epilepsy Behav. 2003;4(5):496-9.
4. Tamilia E, Madsen JR, Grant PE, Pearl PL, Papadelis C. Current and emerging potential of magnetoencephalography in the detection and localization of high-frequency oscillations in epilepsy. Front Neurol. 2017;8:14.
5. Smith SJM, Fisher RS. The minimum standards for long-term video-EEG monitoring in epilepsy. Epilepsia. 2020;61(8):1537-45.
6. Beniczky S, Tatum WO, Blumenfeld H, Stefan H, Mani J, Maillard L, et al. Seizure semiology: ILAE glossary of terms and their significance. Epilepsia. 2022;63(6):1251-62.
7. Baumgartner C, Koren JP, Britto-Arias M, Zoche L, Pirker S. Presurgical epilepsy evaluation and epilepsy surgery. F1000Research. 2019;8(F1000 Faculty Rev):1818.
8. Wiebe S, Blume WT, Girvin JP, Eliasziw M. A randomized, controlled trial of surgery for temporal-lobe epilepsy. N Engl J Med. 2001; 345(5):311-8.
9. Bernasconi A, Cendes F, Theodore WH, Gill RS, Federico P, Ryvlin P, et al. Recommendations for the use of structural magnetic resonance imaging in the care of patients with epilepsy: A consensus report from the International League Against Epilepsy Neuroimaging Task Force. Epilepsia. 2019;60(11):1054-68.
10. Chandra PS, Tripathi M. Epilepsy surgery: recommendations for India. Ann Indian Acad Neurol. 2010;13(2):87-93.
11. Malhotra V, Chandra SP, Dash D, Garg A, Tripathi M, Bal CS, et al. A screening tool to identify surgical candidates with drug refractory epilepsy in a resource limited settings. Epilepsy Res. 2016;121:14-20.
12. Vakharia VN, Duncan JS, Witt JA, Elger CE, Staba R, Engel J Jr. Getting the best outcomes from epilepsy surgery. Epilepsy Behav. 2018;88:24-34.
13. O'Brien TJ, So EL, Mullan BP, Hauser MF, Brinkmann BH, Bohnen NI, et al. Subtraction ictal SPECT co-registered to MRI improves clinical usefulness of SPECT in localizing the surgical seizure focus. Neurology. 1998;50(2):445-54.
14. Chandra PS, Vaghania G, Bal CS, Tripathi M, Kuruwale N, Arora A, et al. Role of concordance between ictal-subtracted SPECT and PET in predicting long-term outcomes after epilepsy surgery. Epilepsy Res. 2014;108(10):1782-9.
15. Kaur K, Garg A, Tripathi M, Chandra SP, Singh G, Viswanathan V, et al. Comparative contribution of magnetoencephalography (MEG) and single-photon emission computed tomography (SPECT) in pre-operative localization for epilepsy surgery: A prospective blinded study. Seizure. 2021;86: 181-8.
16. Tripathi M, Kaur K, Ramanujam B, Viswanathan V, Bharti K, Singh G, et al. Diagnostic added value of interictal magnetic source imaging in presurgical evaluation of persons with epilepsy: A prospective blinded study. Eur J Neurol. 2021;28(9):2940-51.
17. Chandra PS, Doddamani R, Girishan S, Samala R, Agrawal M, Garg A, et al. Robotic thermocoagulative hemispherotomy: concept, feasibility, outcomes, and safety of a new "bloodless" technique. J Neurosurg Pediatr. 2021;27(6):688-99.
18. Chandra PS, Bal C, Garg A, Gaikwad S, Prasad K, Sharma BS, et al. Surgery for medically intractable epilepsy due to postinfectious etiologies. Epilepsia. 2010;51(6):1097-100.
19. Ahmad FU, Tripathi M, Padma MV, Gaikwad S, Gupta A, Bal CS, et al. Health-related quality of life using QOLIE-31: before and after epilepsy surgery a prospective study at a tertiary care center. Neurol India. 2007;55(4):343-8.
20. Dwivedi R, Ramanujam B, Chandra PS, Sapra S, Gulati S, Kalaivani M, et al. Surgery for drug-resistant epilepsy in children. N Engl J Med. 2017;377(17):1639-47.
21. Ben-Menachem E, Revesz D, Simon BJ, Silberstein S. Surgically implanted and non-invasive vagus nerve stimulation: A review of efficacy, safety and tolerability. Eur J Neurol. 2015;22(9):1260-8.
22. Curatolo P, Bombardieri R, Jozwiak S. Tuberous sclerosis. Lancet. 2008;372(9639):657-68.
23. Chandra SP, Kurwale NS, Chibber SS, Banerji J, Dwivedi R, Garg A, et al. Endoscopic-assisted (Through a Mini Craniotomy) corpus callosotomy

combined with anterior, hippocampal, and posterior commissurotomy in Lennox–Gastaut syndrome: A pilot study to establish its safety and efficacy. Neurosurgery. 2016;78(5):743-51.

24. Zangiabadi N, Ladino LD, Sina F, Orozco-Hernández JP, Carter A, Téllez-Zenteno JF. Deep brain stimulation and drug-resistant epilepsy: A review of the literature. Front Neurol. 2019;10:601.

25. Sun FT, Morrell MJ. The RNS System: responsive cortical stimulation for the treatment of refractory partial epilepsy. Expert Rev Med Devices. 2014;11(6):563-72.

26. DeGiorgio CM, Fanselow EE, Schrader LM, Cook IA. Trigeminal nerve stimulation: seminal animal and human studies for epilepsy and depression. Neurosurg Clin N Am. 2011;22(4):449-56.

27. Li Y, Li L, Pan W. Repetitive transcranial magnetic stimulation (rTMS) modulates hippocampal structural synaptic plasticity in rats. Physiol Res. 2019;68(1):99-105.

28. Tekturk P, Erdogan ET, Kurt A, Vanli-Yavuz EN, Ekizoglu E, Kocagoncu E, et al. The effect of transcranial direct current stimulation on seizure frequency of patients with mesial temporal lobe epilepsy with hippocampal sclerosis. Clin Neurol Neurosurg. 2016;149:27-32.

29. Parihar J, Agrawal M, Samala R, Chandra PS, Tripathi M. Role of neuromodulation for treatment of drug-resistant epilepsy. Neurol India. 2020;68(Supplement):S249-58.

30. Sourbron J, Klinkenberg S, van Kuijk SMJ, Lagae L, Lambrechts D, Braakman HMH, et al. Ketogenic diet for the treatment of pediatric epilepsy: review and meta-analysis. Child's Nerv Syst. 2020;36(6):1099-109.

31. Manral M, Tripathi S, Rawat D, Tripathi M. Modified Atkins diet in adolescents and adults with drug resistant epilepsy: A systematic review and meta-analysis. J Epilepsy Res. 2024;14(1):1-8.

32. Manral M, Dwivedi R, Gulati S, Kaur K, Nehra A, Pandey RM, et al. Safety, efficacy, and tolerability of modified Atkins diet in persons with drug-resistant epilepsy: A randomized controlled trial. Neurology. 2023;100(13):e1376-85.

Neurostimulation in Epilepsy

Siby Gopinath, Rutul Shah, Abhishek Gohel

ABSTRACT

Epilepsy affects over seven crore people worldwide, including 1.2 crore in India. Despite advancements in antiseizure medications, about 70% of patients achieve seizure control, leaving 30% requiring alternative treatments. Although surgical resection or ablative procedures offer seizure freedom rates of 40–90%, a significant number of patients are either ineligible for surgery or continue to experience seizures. Neurostimulation therapies, such as vagal nerve stimulation (VNS), deep brain stimulation (DBS), and responsive neurostimulation (RNS), provide viable options for these patients. These procedures target specific brain circuits to modulate dysfunctional networks, offering another treatment avenue.

Vagal nerve stimulation is used as an adjunct therapy for both children and adults, modulating thalamocortical circuits through the vagus afferent network to reduce seizures in about 50% of patients. RNS utilizes a closed-loop system that records intracranial electroencephalogram (EEG) patterns to activate stimulation at appropriate times to prevent seizures. It is particularly effective for seizures originating in the eloquent cortex and multifocal seizure onsets. DBS targets the anterior and centromedian nuclei of the thalamus, with the anterior nucleus treating focal and secondarily generalized drug-resistant epilepsy (DRE), and the centromedian nucleus addressing generalized epilepsies like Lennox–Gastaut syndrome (LGS).

The benefits of stimulation tend to increase over time, with seizure frequency reductions typically around 40% initially, improving to 50–69% over several years. In this chapter, we explore the application of electrical stimulation in epilepsy, potential targets, mechanisms of neuromodulation and seizure control, and clinical evidence.

Keywords: Neuromodulation, DBS, VNS, RNS, Refractory epilepsy, Epilepsy surgery.

"What we know is a drop, what we don't know is an ocean."

—*Sir Issac Newton*

INTRODUCTION

Epilepsy affects over 7 crore people worldwide, including 1.2 crore in India. Epilepsy impacts various aspects of life, and the risk of sudden unexpected death in epilepsy (SUDEP) is 23 times higher for patients living with epilepsy.[1,2] Despite over 30 antiseizure medications available, only 70% of patients achieve seizure control, leaving 30% needing nonmedical treatments like surgery.[3] These procedures have long waiting times and effectiveness drops below 50% after 10 years.[4]

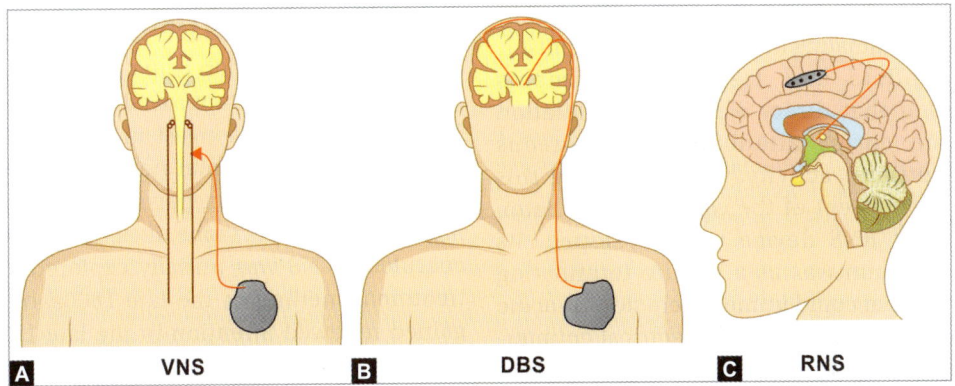

FIGS. 1A TO C: Illustrative comparison of neurostimulation techniques for epilepsy treatment. This figure demonstrates the placement and pathways of VNS in part A, DBS in part B, and RNS in part C. (A) The VNS device setup includes an electrode with three helical contacts connected to a subclavicular implantable pulse generator, illustrating its application; (B) DBS system features depth electrodes connected to a subclavicular implantable pulse generator, highlighting its use in neurostimulation therapy; and (C) RNS configuration with depth electrodes, cortical strips, and a cranial implantable pulse generator, underscoring its role in managing drug-resistant epilepsy.

(DBS: deep brain stimulation; RNS: responsive neurostimulation; VNS: vagus nerve stimulation)

Source: Modified from Gouveia FV, Warsi NM, Suresh H, Matin R, Ibrahim GM. Neurostimulation treatments for epilepsy: deep brain stimulation, responsive neurostimulation, and vagus nerve stimulation. Neurotherapeutics. 2024;21(3):e00308.

Success depends on accurately identifying the epileptogenic zone, and there is a small risk of irreversible neurological damage.

Neurostimulation devices, such as vagal nerve stimulation (VNS), deep brain stimulation (DBS), and responsive neurostimulation (RNS), offer another treatment option by implanting electrodes in the brain to modulate dysfunctional circuits. VNS and DBS are approved in India and use either open-loop or closed-loop stimulation paradigms **(Figs. 1A to C)**.[5]

■ MECHANISM OF ACTION IN NEUROMODULATION THROUGH ELECTRICAL STIMULATION

The mechanisms of neuromodulatory effects of electrical stimulation, such as DBS, are complex and not fully understood. Initially, DBS was thought to inhibit neural activity similarly to ablative techniques, creating a reversible, functional lesion.[6] Electrical stimulation impacts neural circuits based on amplitude, frequency, pulse width, and polarity, potentially blocking or substituting abnormal neural signals with therapeutic patterns.[7]

Mechanisms such as depolarization blockade, synaptic inhibition, synaptic depression, and disruption of pathological network activity explain its effects on neurological disorders.[8-10] Therapies like VNS and DBS affect neurochemical interactions and influence gene and protein expression. Low-frequency stimulation modifies adenosine receptor gene expression, contributing to its anticonvulsant properties. VNS alters neurotransmitters and hormones in cerebrospinal fluid, enhancing epilepsy management. Long-term electrical stimulation leads to adaptive neurochemical and synaptic changes, resulting in progressive improvement in treatment outcomes.[11] It operates through an extensive vagus afferent network connecting the brainstem to various cerebral structures. This network helps desynchronize epileptiform activities, particularly within the gamma-frequency band, modulating thalamocortical circuits.

Penfield and Jasper's experiments showed that direct electrical stimulation of the cortex attenuated spontaneous epileptiform activity.[12] Extrapolating this on the concept of the cardiac defibrillator, the first RNS device was developed. Its primary aim was as a seizure-terminating device, that could immediately stop an acute seizure through targeted electrical counter-stimulation of the spiking, which occurred during ictal activity in the brain.[13] In addition to the advantage of acute seizure termination, patients who underwent RNS were also found to have long-term benefits. Due to chronic stimulation, differential plasticity was developed in the functional network connectivity, which contributed to an overall better long-term clinical outcome.[14]

■ VAGAL NERVE STIMULATION

Vagal nerve stimulation is the first electrical stimulation therapy approved for epilepsy. The vagus nerve, the longest and most widely distributed of all cranial nerves, connects extensively to various parts of the brain, including the dorsal raphe nucleus and locus coeruleus. VNS was initially explored as a treatment method in the late 1800s, but it gained renewed attention in the late 1980s for managing refractory epilepsy. Since then, VNS has also been approved for treating severe obesity, and depression unresponsive to other treatments, in addition to its use in managing refractory epilepsy.[15] In June 2017, the United States Food and Drug Administration (US FDA) extended approval to include patients aged 4 years and older with refractory seizures **(Fig. 2)**.

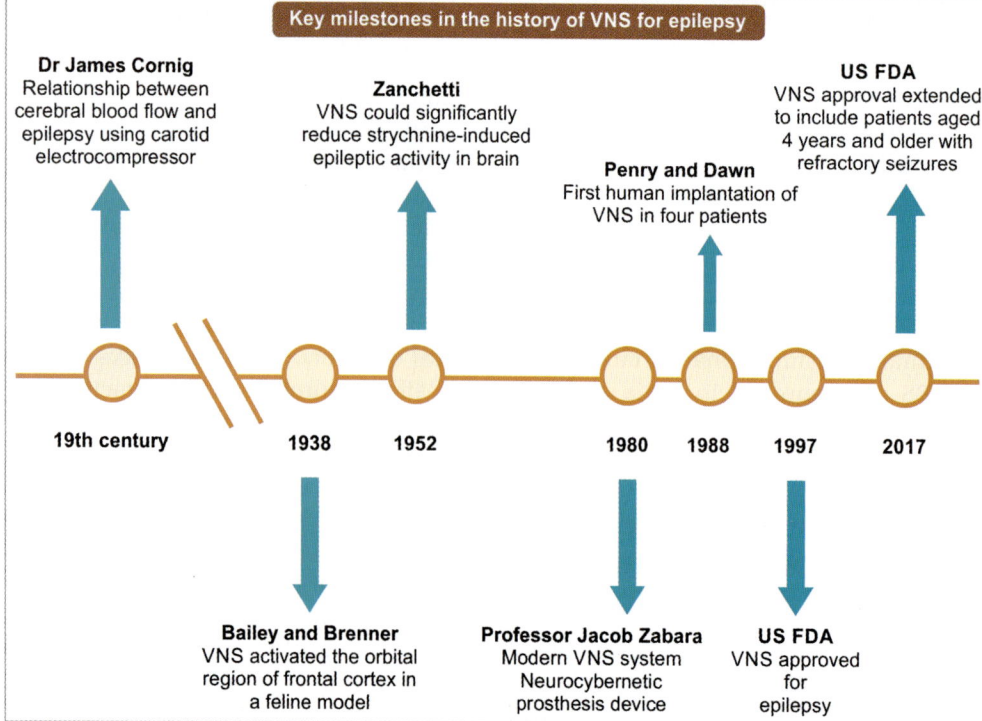

FIG. 2: Timeline of key milestones in developing and implementing VNS for epilepsy. This timeline illustrates significant historical events from the 19th century through 2017, detailing the evolution of VNS from conceptual studies to FDA approvals for treating epilepsy.
(US FDA: United States Food and Drug Administration; VNS: vagal nerve stimulation)

Method

Vagal nerve stimulation involves the implantation of a neurocybernetic prosthesis, which includes bipolar leads coiled around the left vagus nerve. The left side is chosen because stimulating the right vagus nerve can cause bradycardia by affecting the sinoatrial node. These electrodes are connected to an implantable, multiprogrammable pulse generator placed subcutaneously below the clavicle. The system is chronically stimulated using a programming wand, and the generator's battery life ranges from 3–5 years. Additionally, the patient or caregiver is provided with a handheld magnet, which can deliver extra stimulation at the onset of an aura or seizure, or to switch off the system, for example, during public speaking or during magnetic resonance imaging (MRI).

Clinical Evidence for Vagus Nerve Stimulation

Several randomized control trials (RCTs) support evidence for the efficacy of VNS in treating refractory epilepsy.

In these trials, patients who were followed up over time showed improved VNS efficacy with prolonged use. The EO5 trial found a 45% mean seizure reduction at 12 months for 195 patients, while the EO3 trial reported a 52% reduction at 18 months for 67 patients **(Table 1)**.[16,17]

TABLE 1: Comparative analysis of EO3 and EO5 trials on vagus nerve stimulation (VNS) in patients with refractory epilepsy. This table outlines the methodologies, parameters, and outcomes of two multicenter, prospective, double-blind, randomized controlled trials investigating the efficacy of VNS in reducing seizure frequency among patients with refractory epilepsy.[16,17]

Study name	EO3 Trial	EO5 Trial
Type	Multicenter, prospective double-blind, randomized parallel design	Multicenter, prospective double-blind, randomized parallel design
Participants	Patients with refractory epilepsy; at least 6 seizures in the past 30 days; seizure-free interval not exceeding 14 days; AED levels variation <20%	Patients with refractory focal epilepsy; at least 6 seizures in the past 30 days; seizure-free interval not exceeding 21 days; stable AED regimen
Baseline period	12 weeks of monitoring seizure type, frequency, and antiseizure drugs	12–16 weeks of monitoring seizure records, adverse events, and medications
Procedure	Implantation of vagal nerve stimulation device around the left vagus nerve, connected to a subcutaneous generator below the clavicle	Implantation of stimulating electrodes around the left vagus nerve, connected to a subcutaneous generator below the clavicle
Stimulation start	2 weeks postimplantation	2 weeks postimplantation
Randomization	High-stimulation (HS) group and low-stimulation (LS) group	High-stimulation (HS) group and low -stimulation (IS) group
HS group parameters	• *Current:* 0.25–3 mA • *Frequency:* 20-50 Hz • *Pulse duration:* 500 μs • *On period:* 30–90 sec • *Off period:* 5–10 minutes	• *Current:* Up to 3.5 mA • *Frequency:* 30 Hz *Pulse duration:* 500 μs • *On period:* 30 sec every 5 minutes

Continued

Continued

Study name	EO3 Trial	EO5 Trial
LS Group parameters	• *Current:* 0.25–2.75 mA • *Frequency:* 1–2 Hz • *Pulse duration:* 130 μs • *On period:* 30 sec • *Off period:* 60–180 minutes	• *Frequency:* 1 Hz • *Pulse duration:* 130 μs • *On period:* 30 sec every 3 hours
Manual activation	HS group could manually activate for 30 seconds stimulation at seizure onset	HS group could manually activate for 30 seconds stimulation at seizure onset
Assessment period	12–16 weeks postrandomization	12–16 weeks postrandomization; eligible for open treatment extension phase
Participants randomized	125	254 (196 analyzed)
Participants completed	114	196
Outcome (HS vs. LS)	*Seizure reduction:* HS (−24.5%) vs. IS (−6.1%); $p = 0.01$	*Seizure reduction:* HS (−27.9%) versus LS (−15.2%); $p = 0.04$
Baseline comparison	• HS: Significant reduction ($p < 0.01$, 95% CI, 14.1% to −34.9%) • LS: Not significant ($p = 0.21$, 95% CI, 3.6% to −15.8%)	Both groups achieved statistical significance; HS group had a greater reduction in seizures
Seizure freedom	None in HS group achieved seizure freedom	1 patient in HS group was completely seizure-free
Adverse events	<5% of study group; common: hoarseness/tremulous voice, throat pain, cough, dyspnea, paresthesias, and muscle pain	-

(AED: antiepileptic drugs; CI: confidence interval)

According to the 2013 American Academy of Neurology (AAN) guideline update, VNS resulted in a >50% seizure reduction in 55% of 470 children with refractory epilepsy and 55% of 113 patients with LGS. The update also noted VNS's efficacy in improving mood problems in adults and increased efficacy over time.[18]

An analysis of around 400 patients who were followed up for 5 years reported around 55% reduction in seizures and a long-term follow-up (10 years) of 65 of the initial cohort reported close to 75% reduction in seizures.[19,20] Similarly, an analysis of around 3,000 patients and a registry of around 5,500 patients suggested that close to 60% of patients had more than 50% reduction at 2-4 years and 8% of those were seizure-free.[21] The Patient Outcome Registry also detected that those patients had a better quality of life including improvement in mood. This led to FDA approval of VNS in 2005 for depression cases, which were refractory to medications.[22] On-demand VNS automatically provides stimulation in response to changes in heart rate, eliminating the need for a voluntary magnetic swipe.[23]

A large number of patients with epilepsy experience ictal tachycardia. Responsive VNS (rVNS) implements an algorithm that utilizes heart rate as a parameter for stimulation.

A mode of VNS, AutoStim was first clinically evaluated in a multicentric study in Europe as well as in the US where around 3/4th of seizures experienced ictal tachycardia. Automatic stimulation treated 35% of the seizures, and of these, 61% were terminated by the automatic stimulation. At 1 year follow-up, half of the patients had improvement in seizure severity and quality of life. Almost 30% of the patients who replaced traditional VNS with AutoStim had a reduction in seizures.[24]

Dosing Vagus Nerve Stimulation

Vagus nerve stimulation is an electroceutical therapy with dosing adjusted through current settings to find a therapeutic level tolerable for the patient. Stimulation starts 2 weeks after implantation at a current of 0.25 mA and is increased by 0.25 fortnightly to reach a target of 1.5–2.25 mA. The pulse width is 250 µs and the frequency is 20 Hz.[25]

The duty cycle, the percentage of time VNS remains active, is 10% with 30 seconds on and 5 minutes off. Reducing the off time to 1.1 minutes or less can benefit patients with seizures at lower currents.

The current is 0.25 mA higher in magnet mode than in normal mode. In AutoStim mode, the current applied is 0.125 mA greater than the standard level, where it compares the heart rate over the last 10 seconds with the preceding 5 minutes. The range of automatic stimulation threshold is 20–70% increase in heart rate. **Table 2** summarizes the common side effects of VNS and its management.

■ DEEP BRAIN STIMULATION

Deep Brain Stimulation Targets

Anterior Nucleus of Thalamus

In 1937, James W Papez introduced the concept of the Papez circuit, a neural loop that connects the hippocampus with the mammillary bodies, anterior nucleus of thalamus (ANT), and cingulate cortex, ultimately circling back to the hippocampus. This circuit is connected to the brain's frontal, temporal, and parietal regions, with evidence supporting its presence in patients with hippocampal sclerosis.[27]

The ANT is the only FDA-approved thalamic nucleus for epilepsy treatment, specifically targeted for DBS. It connects to

TABLE 2: Overview of common side effects, prevalence, and management strategies for vagal nerve stimulation (VNS) in patients.[26]

Side effect	Prevalence	Symptoms/effects	Management
Laryngeal and pharyngeal dysfunction	Up to 60% of cases	Hoarseness, voice alteration, dysphagia, dyspnea, or cough	Reduce frequency of stimulation, use magnet during meals for dysphagia
Cardiac bradyarrhythmia	More common in adults	No significant events reported in studies	No significant events reported in studies
Sleep apnea	Unfavorable impact on upper airway	Increased severity of OSA or new-onset OSA	Use CPAP, modify stimulation parameters
MRI considerations	MRI conditional	Special precautions needed	Turn off device during MRI, check programming after, and use head coil

(CPAP: continuous positive airway pressure; MRI: magnetic resonance imaging; OSA: obstructive sleep apnea)

the limbic system and various brain regions, serving as the primary hub of the limbic thalamus due to its extensive connectivity **(Fig. 3)**.

Advantages of targeting the ANT:
- Small size
- Extensive projections to limbic structures, which are connected to the neocortex
- *Accessibility:* Not near the vascular structures

Pioneering Work and Clinical Trials

The DBS for epilepsy was pioneered by Irving Cooper.[28] The SANTÉ trial, a multicenter, double-blind RCT by Fisher et al. in 2010, involved 110 patients with refractory epilepsy. Patients received DBS or no stimulation for 3 months, followed by 9 months of unblinded stimulation. The stimulation group had a 29% seizure reduction compared to controls. At 2 years, the group had a 56% median reduction in seizure frequency, with 54% experiencing a 50% reduction, and 14 patients were seizure-free for at least 6 months. A 10-year follow-up showed a 75% median seizure reduction, with no significant cognitive symptoms or serious adverse events, indicating stable long-term efficacy and safety.[28,29]

Other studies show similar results to SANTÉ, with reports indicating that DBS coupled with an RNS system near the seizure focus can result in at least a 50% seizure reduction.[30] Case reports support the efficacy of ANT DBS in super-refractory status epilepticus.

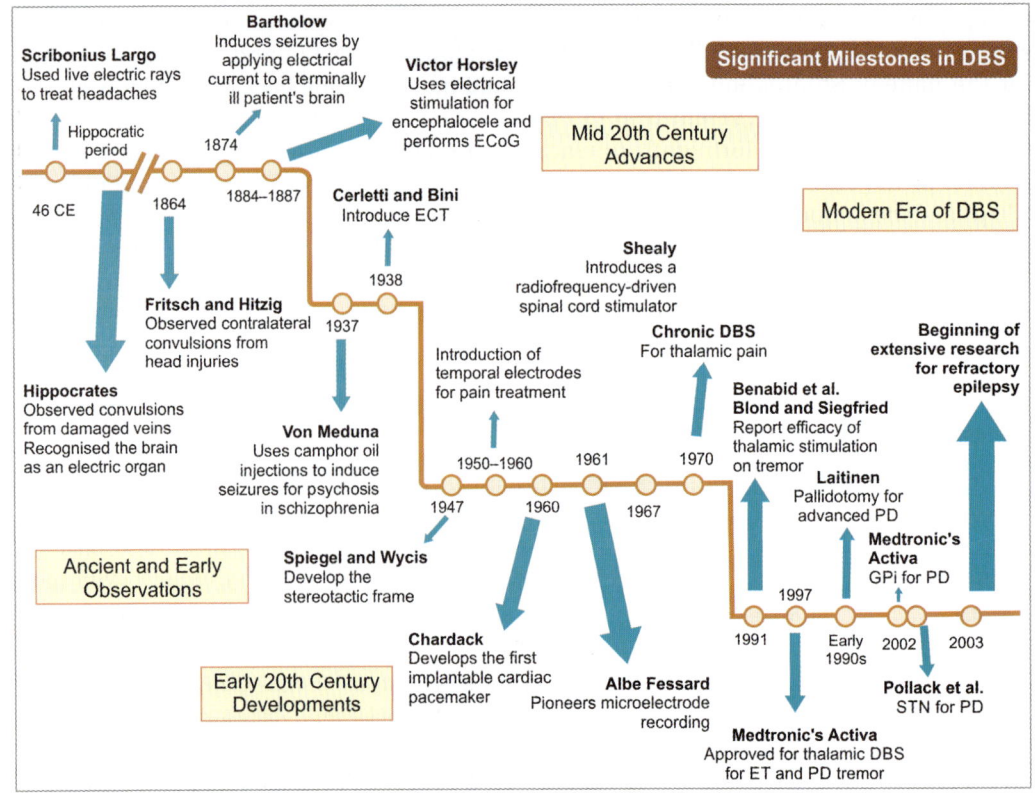

FIG. 3: Timeline of DBS: A historical overview.

(DBS: deep brain stimulation; ET: essential tremor; ECT: electroconvulsive therapy; ECoG: electrocorticography; PD: Parkinson's disease; STN: subthalamic nucleus; GPi: globus pallidus interna)

Stimulation Parameters

Neurostimulation involves many parameters:
- Electrode configuration
- Target of electrode implantation
- The stimulation frequency
- The pulse width of the stimulus
- The current used
- Bipolar versus referential stimulation polarities

Methods of Stimulation

These include the following:
- Continuous
- Intermittent stimulation
- Responsive stimulation

Note that there are no definite guidelines for the selection of specific stimulation parameters, and it often involves a trial-and-error method.

In the SANTÉ trial, the setup of the stimulating electrodes involved positioning the central-most contact in each anterior nucleus as the cathode. At the same time, the stimulator case acted as the anode. Stimulation began 1 month after implantation.

The stimulation parameters:
- *Current:* 5 V
- *Pulse width:* 90 microseconds
- *Stimulation frequency:* 145 Hz
- The stimulation operated in a cycling mode, with an "on" time of 1 minute and an "off" time of 5 minutes **(Flowchart 1)**.

Clinical Surveys

Two surveys provide insights into prevalent stimulation parameters for ANT-DBS. The US survey found that most parameters aligned with the SANTÉ trial, except for lower initial amplitude, with adjustments made based on efficacy and side effects.[31] The European survey preferred monopolar stimulation and SANTÉ parameters, with variability in amplitude.[32] Side effects were managed by adjusting stimulation settings or using bilevel stimulation at night.

Centromedian Nucleus

Stimulation of the ANT is effective for focal epilepsy, especially temporal lobe epilepsy, while the *centromedian nucleus* (CMN) is gaining evidence for treating generalized

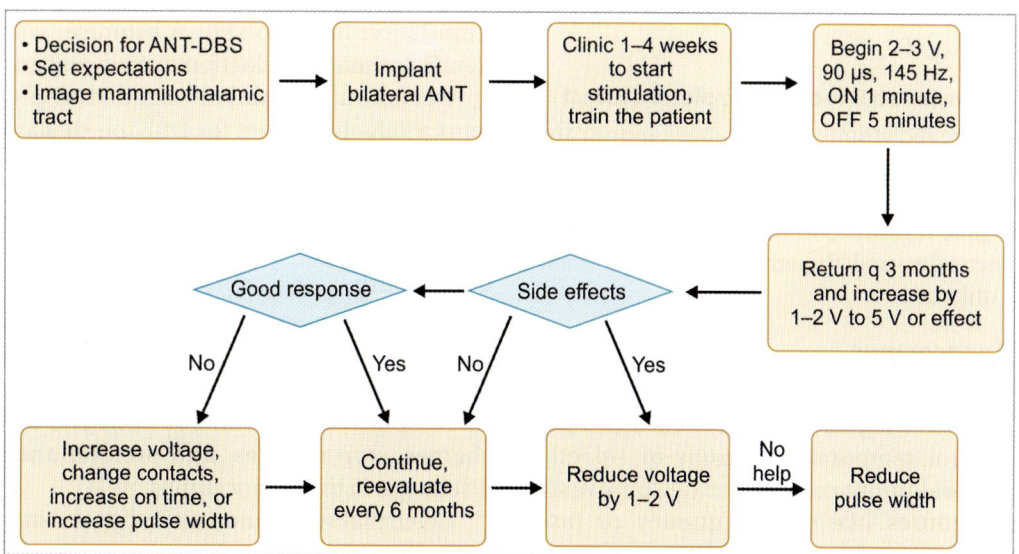

FLOWCHART 1: Decision-making flowchart for anterior nucleus of the thalamus deep brain stimulation (ANT-DBS) Management.
Source: Modified from Fasano et al. (2021).

epilepsies and multifocal seizures. Located in the caudal part of the intralaminar thalamic nuclei, the CMN is connected to the reticular nucleus of the thalamus and is a potential target for neuromodulation.[33]

Early reports on CMN stimulation's efficacy for generalized epilepsy were published by Velasco et al. in 1987.[34] Subsequent studies supported its benefits. Recent studies, such as the one conducted by Cukiert et al., demonstrated a 90% response rate, with over a 50% reduction in the frequency of seizures with significant improvement in attention.[35]

The ESTEL trial is the first double-blind, RCT that was a placebo-controlled study of DBS of CMN in adult patients of LGS. Results showed that 50% of the treatment group achieved at least a 50% reduction in seizures compared to around 20% in the control group. Around 90% of the patients had a significant reduction in electrographic seizures.[36]

A related study by Valentín et al. found significant seizure reduction in generalized epilepsy but less efficacy in focal epilepsy, supporting CMN stimulation as a promising treatment for refractory generalized epilepsy.[37]

Implantation Effect or Microlesion Effect

Seizure reduction occurs within 1 month after implantation in about 20% of cases, peaking at 2-3 months, even before the stimulation begins, regardless of the target or number of electrodes used, though the exact mechanism is unknown.

Hippocampus

The hippocampus is a common target for DRE, with high seizure freedom rates post anterior temporal lobectomy or selective amygdalohippocampectomy. Noninvasive procedures like radiofrequency or laser ablation are also effective. However, hippocampal resection may not be feasible for dominant medial temporal lobe epilepsy with preserved verbal memory, bilateral medial temporal lobe epilepsy, or relapsed seizures postsurgery.

Animal studies show that electrical stimulation of hippocampal slices can reduce seizures significantly. Human trials by Velasco et al. on hippocampal stimulation showed significant seizure reduction and decreased interictal spikes, with long-lasting antiepileptic effects without language and memory adverse effects.[38]

In an 18-month follow-up, Velasco et al. found that four out of nine patients were seizure-free, with significant seizure reduction in patients without hippocampal sclerosis. Boon's group reported a 8.5 years follow-up where 6 out of 11 patients had over a 90% reduction in seizures, with 3 becoming seizure-free.[39] Boëx et al. documented significant seizure reduction in patients with contacts near the subiculum.[40] A randomized, double-blind study by Cukiert et al. showed 50% seizure freedom in the active group, with better responses in patients with hippocampal sclerosis.[41]

Noninvasive transcranial direct cortical stimulation has also shown promise, with significant seizure reduction in most patients.

Overall, hippocampal stimulation presents a valuable option for DRE, particularly when resection or ablation is not feasible, demonstrating significant seizure reduction with minimal cognitive impact.

Cerebellum

The cerebellum was one of the earliest targets for DBS in epilepsy, starting in the 1950s. Animal studies demonstrated that cerebellar stimulation could influence epileptic discharges, stop seizures, and prolong afterdischarges in the hippocampus.[42]

Cerebellar stimulation works by inhibiting thalamic activity through the Purkinje cells' output, which connects to the cortex and brainstem. Early human trials in the 70s and 80s showed mixed results, with some improvement in seizure control but also notable issues like lead migration, infection, and mechanical failure.

Interest in cerebellar stimulation waned until a 2005 trial by Velasco showed a 33% seizure reduction at 3 months and further improvements at 6 months. However, small sample sizes, conflicting results, and high complication rates have kept cerebellar stimulation a questionable treatment for intractable epilepsy.[43]

Midbrain and Subthalamic Nucleus

The substantia nigra and subthalamic nucleus (STN) have been explored as DBS targets in epilepsy through experimental animal models, which showed that increasing gamma-aminobutyric acid (GABA) availability in the midbrain could block seizures. The substantia nigra is critical for preventing the propagation of generalized seizures.

The STN stimulation works by inhibiting the substantia nigra pars reticulata, which decreases its firing and disinhibits the dorsal midbrain anticonvulsant zone. It also activates the cortico-subthalamic pathway, reducing cortical excitability. Studies, such as Benabid et al. in 2002, reported an 80% seizure reduction over 30 months.[44]

Clinical trials have shown varying degrees of success, with seizure frequency reductions ranging from 42–75% in patients with resistant epilepsy. However, outcomes can vary based on seizure type and individual patient conditions.

Multitarget Deep Brain Stimulation

The SANTÉ trial showed a 75% reduction in seizures with multitarget DBS over 7 years, with the best results for temporal and frontal seizures (70–86%). In patients with parietal, occipital, multifocal, and diffuse seizures, the reduction was lower at 31%.

For cases with poor outcomes, DBS targeting two to three distinct nuclei was performed. This approach included at least one well-researched target such as the ANT or CMN, in addition to targets like the pulvinar, medial dorsal nucleus, or STN. 8 patients underwent this approach, and all with over 6 months of follow-up achieved at least a 50% reduction in seizures without serious adverse events.[45]

New Generation of Sensing-enabled Deep Brain Stimulation

New sensing-enabled DBS devices can detect changes in local field potentials at the implantation sites, but clinical translation remains incomplete as they can not yet adjust therapy based on these changes. Further research is needed to identify reliable biomarkers of seizure activity and develop a truly closed-loop system.

■ RESPONSIVE NEUROSTIMULATION

Responsive neurostimulation is a neuromodulatory treatment approved by the US FDA in 2013 for the treatment of DRE. RNS is the first implantable, brain-responsive neurostimulator approved as an adjunctive treatment for drug-refractory focal epilepsy. RNS being a closed-loop system, continuously tracks the electrical activity at the epileptogenic foci and it delivers stimulation only when an ictal graph previously identified and set by the treating physician is detected.

The stimulation in RNS consists of pulses of current provided through a combination of the electrodes. After the implantation, the physician programs the stimulation pathway and sets the parameters like current magnitude (in mA), frequency, duration

of burst, and pulse width **(Fig. 4)**. The stimulation settings used in various studies are mentioned below:
- *Frequency:* 100–200 Hz
- *Current:* 1.5–3 mA
- *Pulse width:* 160 microseconds
- *Pulse duration:* 100–200 milliseconds

Usually, the device detects ~600–2,000 ictal activities per day following which the stimulation occurs. This amounts to around 5–6 minutes of stimulation daily. Considering this scenario, the battery life of the device is around 8.5 years.

Clinical Evidence for Responsive Neurostimulation

The majority of evidence available for RNS is because of clinical trials that involved the implantation of around 250 patients across 3 trials. 2 of the trials had data from 2 years while 1 of them was a long-term treatment study (7 years).[46-49]

In a pivotal trial by Morrell et al., 191 patients were assessed for the safety and feasibility of RNS. At 5 months, the control group had a close to 10% reduction in seizure frequency while the implanted patients showed around 40% reduction in seizures, with a 25% reduction even before stimulation began. During the open-label follow-up, median seizure reduction improved from 44% at 1 year to 75% at 9 years. The outcomes were consistent across different implantation sites and unaffected by changes in antiepileptic drugs.

Adverse Events and Quality of Life

There was no significant difference in adverse events when the stimulated group was compared to the control group. Device-related complications over 2 years included a 3.7% infection rate, 2.6% lead damage, and 3.7% lead displacement.[48,49] The SUDEP was 2.95 per 1,000 patient-years which is much

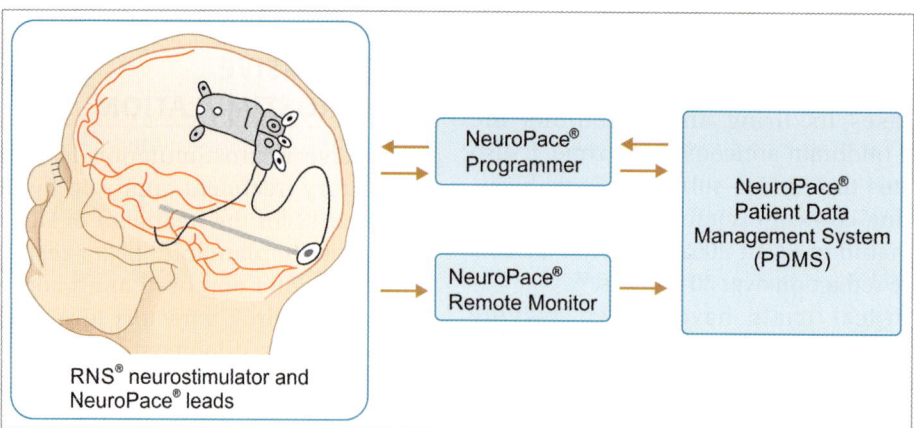

FIG. 4: Comprehensive view of the RNS® neurostimulator system components and connectivity. This diagram presents the RNS® neurostimulator with NeuroPace® leads (including depth and/or cortical strip leads, depending on the target area) implanted in the brain. The system's implantable components—neurostimulator and leads—are crucial for recording and stimulation. The NeuroPace® programmer, interacts directly with the neurostimulator. This programmer is utilized by physicians to adjust the neurostimulator's detection and stimulation settings and to access data recorded by the device. Additionally, the remote monitor, a patient-operated home monitoring device, facilitates the retrieval of data from the neurostimulator to upload to the NeuroPace® patient data management system (PDMS). This centralized database consolidates data from both the programmer and the remote monitor, enabling comprehensive monitoring and management of patient data.

Source: Modified from Skarpaas et al. (2019).

lower than DRE patients who had surgical failure.[50]

Patients experienced better quality of life and cognitive improvements compared to medical treatment, without significant mood or cognitive adverse events.

Insights from Chronic Ambulatory Electrocorticographic Monitoring

Responsive neurostimulation provides access to long-term data on electrocortical events, spanning from days to months. This helps in understanding patient-specific temporal dynamics in epileptiform activity. Chronic electrocorticography (ECoG) recording has demonstrated its efficacy in identifying patients for resection who were initially thought to be nonresectable due to the multifocality in their long term EEG monitoring data.[51]

Thirteen percent of patients in the pivotal trial who were suspected to have bilateral mesial temporal lobe epilepsy were detected to have unilateral seizures when they were on their routine medications in their natural environment.

In cases of mesial temporal lobe epilepsy, it took an average of around 41.6 days of recording to determine that seizures arose bilaterally, which is beyond the usual EMU data recording duration. The chronic electrocorticographic data from RNS could also predict responsiveness to a new antiseizure medication (ASM) treatment and showed that 90% of the patients had circadian periodicities in their electrographic seizures.[52]

■ CONCLUSION

Neurostimulation has been explored as a treatment for epilepsy for over 50 years, with VNS, DBS (targeting the ANT), and RNS being the three modalities approved by the FDA. The efficacy of these treatments is measured by a reduction of >50% in seizure frequency. Achieving seizure control is crucial, as the quality of life for patients with epilepsy largely depends on seizure freedom. Despite the long history of electrical stimulation, the exact mechanisms of action remain rudimentary. Understanding these mechanisms could enhance our knowledge of network dynamics, target selection, and stimulation parameters, ultimately leading to more tailored and effective treatments.

Technological innovations, such as more predictable and directed stimulation, steerable stimulation, and closed-loop systems, offer promise for improving outcomes, reducing device longevity issues, and enhancing tolerability. Additionally, applying stimulation indirectly to deep nuclei like the ANT and CMN within the epileptogenic network can selectively modulate different cell populations. Advances in structural imaging, such as diffusion tensor imaging (DTI), functional imaging like the default mode network, and virtual epileptic brain modeling, could further refine neurostimulation techniques.

The results of pivotal trials show promising seizure reduction rates over time: VNS achieved a 41% reduction at both 2 and 3 years, DBS targeting the ANT achieved up to a 56% reduction at 2 years, and RNS showed a 60% reduction by the 3rd year. As we continue to progress, these advancements may pave the way for more effective and personalized treatment options for epilepsy patients.

"Healing is not an event, it's a journey."
—**Anonymous**

REFERENCES

1. Amudhan S, Gururaj G, Satishchandra P. Epilepsy in India I: Epidemiology and public health. Ann Indian Acad Neurol. 2015;18(3):263-77.
2. Mesraoua B, Tomson T, Brodie M, Asadi-Pooya AA. Sudden unexpected death in epilepsy (SUDEP): Definition, epidemiology, and significance of education. Epilepsy Behav. 2022;132:108742.
3. Wiebe S, Jette N. Pharmacoresistance and the role of surgery in difficult to treat epilepsy. Nat Rev Neurol. 2012;8(12):669-77.
4. De Tisi J, Bell GS, Peacock JL, McEvoy AW, Harkness WF, Sander JW, et al. The long-term outcome of adult epilepsy surgery, patterns of seizure remission, and relapse: A cohort study. Lancet. 2011;378(9800):1388-95.
5. Ryvlin P, Rheims S, Hirsch LJ, Sokolov A, Jehi L. Neuromodulation in epilepsy: State-of-the-art approved therapies. Lancet Neurol. 2021;20(12):1038-47.
6. Boon P, Raedt R, de Herdt V, Wyckhuys T, Vonck K. Electrical stimulation for the treatment of epilepsy. Neurotherapeutics. 2009;6(2):218-27.
7. Gross RE, Laxpati NG, McMahon JT. Electrical Stimulation for Epilepsy (VNS, DBS, and RNS). [online]. Available from https://www.clinicalkey.fr/#!/content/book/3-s2.0-B9780323661928001002?scrollTo=%23hl0001889 [Last accessed August, 2024].
8. Dostrovsky JO, Levy R, Wu JP, Hutchison WD, Tasker RR, Lozano AM. Microstimulation-induced inhibition of neuronal firing in human globus pallidus. J Neurophysiol. 2000;84(1):570-4.
9. Beurrier C, Bioulac B, Audin J, Hammond C. High-frequency stimulation produces a transient blockade of voltage-gated currents in subthalamic neurons. J Neurophysiol. 2001;85(4):1351-6.
10. Jaseja H. EEG-desynchronization as the major mechanism of anti-epileptic action of vagal nerve stimulation in patients with intractable seizures: Clinical neurophysiological evidence. Med Hypotheses. 2010;74(5):855-6.
11. Jahanshahi A, Mirnajafi-Zadeh J, Javan M, Mohammad-Zadeh M, Rohani R. The anti-epileptogenic effect of electrical stimulation at different low frequencies is accompanied with change in adenosine receptors gene expression in rats. Epilepsia. 2009;50(7):1768-79.
12. Penfield W, Jasper H. APA PsycNet Epilepsy and the functional anatomy of the human brain. [online]. Available from https://psycnet.apa.org/record/1955-01377-000 [Last accessed August, 2024].
13. Morrell M. Brain stimulation for epilepsy: Can scheduled or responsive neurostimulation stop seizures? Curr Opin Neurol. 2006;19(2):164-8.
14. Khambhati AN, Shafi A, Rao VR, Chang EF. Long-term brain network reorganization predicts responsive neurostimulation outcomes for focal epilepsy. Sci Transl Med. 2021;13(608).
15. Zabara J. Peripheral control of hypersynchronous discharge in epilepsy. Electroencephalogr Clin Neurophysiol. 1985;61(3):S162.
16. George R, Sonnen A, Upton A, Salinsky M, Ristanovic R, Bergen D, et al.; The Vagus Nerve Stimulation Study Group. A randomized controlled trial of chronic vagus nerve stimulation for treatment of medically intractable seizures. Neurology. 1995;45(2):224-30.
17. Handforth A, DeGiorgio CM, Schachter SC, Uthman BM, Naritoku DK, Tecoma ES, et al. Vagus nerve stimulation therapy for partial-onset seizures: A randomized active-control trial. Neurology. 1998;51(1):48-55.
18. Morris GL, Gloss D, Buchhalter J, Mack KJ, Nickels K, Harden C. Evidence-based guideline update: Vagus nerve stimulation for the treatment of epilepsy: Report of the Guideline Development Subcommittee of the American Academy of Neurology. Neurology. 2013;81(16):1453-9.
19. Elliott RE, Morsi A, Kalhorn SP, Marcus J, Sellin J, Kang M, et al. Vagus nerve stimulation in 436 consecutive patients with treatment-resistant epilepsy: Long-term outcomes and predictors of response. Epilepsy Behav. 2011;20(1):57-63.
20. Elliott RE, Morsi A, Tanweer O, Grobelny B, Geller E, Carlson C, et al. Efficacy of vagus nerve stimulation over time: Review of 65 consecutive patients with treatment-resistant epilepsy treated with VNS >10 years. Epilepsy Behav. 2011;20(3):478-83.
21. Englot DJ, Rolston JD, Wright CW, Hassnain KH, Chang EF. Rates and predictors of seizure freedom with vagus nerve stimulation for intractable epilepsy. Neurosurgery. 2016;79(3):345-53.
22. Englot DJ, Hassnain KH, Rolston JD, Harward SC, Sinha SR, Haglund MM. Quality-of-life metrics with vagus nerve stimulation for epilepsy from provider survey data. Epilepsy Behav. 2017;66:4-9.
23. Fisher RS, Eggleston KS, Wright CW. Vagus nerve stimulation magnet activation for seizures:

A critical review. Acta Neurol Scand. 2015;131(1):1-8.
24. Fisher RS, Afra P, Macken M, Minecan DN, Bagić A, Benbadis SR, et al. Automatic vagus nerve stimulation triggered by ictal tachycardia: Clinical outcomes and device performance–The US E-37 Trial. Neuromodulation. 2016;19(2):188-95.
25. Heck C, Helmers SL, DeGiorgio CM. Vagus nerve stimulation therapy, epilepsy, and device parameters: Scientific basis and recommendations for use. Neurology. 2002;59(6 Suppl 4).
26. Ben-Menachem E. Vagus nerve stimulation, side effects, and long-term safety. J Clin Neurophysiol. 2001;18(5):415-8.
27. Oikawa H, Sasaki M, Tamakawa Y, Kamei A. The circuit of Papez in mesial temporal sclerosis: MRI. Neuroradiology. 2001;43(3):205-10.
28. Fisher R, Salanova V, Witt T, Worth R, Henry T, Gross R, et al. Electrical stimulation of the anterior nucleus of thalamus for treatment of refractory epilepsy. Epilepsia. 2010;51(5):899-908.
29. Salanova V, Sperling MR, Gross RE, Irwin CP, Vollhaber JA, Giftakis JE, et al. The SANTÉ study at 10 years of follow-up: Effectiveness, safety, and sudden unexpected death in epilepsy. Epilepsia. 2021;62(6):1306-17.
30. Herrman H, Egge A, Konglund AE, Ramm-Pettersen J, Dietrichs E, Taubøll E. Anterior thalamic deep brain stimulation in refractory epilepsy: A randomized, double-blinded study. Acta Neurol Scand. 2019;139(3):294-304.
31. Fasano A, Eliashiv D, Herman ST, Lundstrom BN, Polnerow D, Henderson JM, et al. Experience and consensus on stimulation of the anterior nucleus of thalamus for epilepsy. Epilepsia. 2021;62(12):2883-98.
32. Kaufmann E, Bartolomei F, Boon P, Chabardes S, Colon AJ, Eross L, et al. European Expert Opinion on ANT-DBS therapy for patients with drug-resistant epilepsy (a Delphi consensus). Seizure. 2020;81:201-9.
33. Ilyas A, Pizarro D, Romeo AK, Riley KO, Pati S. The centromedian nucleus: Anatomy, physiology, and clinical implications. J Clin Neurosci. 2019;63:1-7.
34. Velasco F, Velasco M, Ogarrio C, Fanghanel G. Electrical stimulation of the centromedian thalamic nucleus in the treatment of convulsive seizures: A preliminary report. Epilepsia. 1987;28(4):421-30.
35. Cukiert A, Cukiert CM, Burattini JA, Mariani PP. Seizure outcome during bilateral, continuous, thalamic centromedian nuclei deep brain stimulation in patients with generalized epilepsy: A prospective, open-label study. Seizure. 2020;81:304-9.
36. Dalic LJ, Warren AEL, Bulluss KJ, Thevathasan W, Roten A, Churilov L, et al. DBS of thalamic centromedian nucleus for Lennox-Gastaut syndrome (ESTEL Trial). Ann Neurol. 2022;91(2):253-67.
37. Valentín A, García Navarrete E, Chelvarajah R, Torres C, Navas M, Vico L, et al. Deep brain stimulation of the centromedian thalamic nucleus for the treatment of generalized and frontal epilepsies. Epilepsia. 2013;54(10):1823-33.
38. Velasco AL, Velasco M, Velasco F, Menes D, Gordon F, Rocha L, et al. Subacute and chronic electrical stimulation of the hippocampus on intractable temporal lobe seizures: Preliminary report. Arch Med Res. 2000;31(3):316-28.
39. Vonck K, Sprengers M, Carrette E, Dauwe I, Miatton M, Meurs A, et al. A decade of experience with deep brain stimulation for patients with refractory medial temporal lobe epilepsy. International journal of neural systems. 2013;23(01):1250034.
40. Boëx C, Seeck M, Vulliémoz S, Rossetti AO, Staedler C, Spinelli L, et al. Chronic deep brain stimulation in mesial temporal lobe epilepsy. Seizure. 2011;20(6):485-90.
41. Cukiert A, Cukiert CM, Burattini JA, Mariani PP, Bezerra DF. Seizure outcome after hippocampal deep brain stimulation in patients with refractory temporal lobe epilepsy: A prospective, controlled, randomized, double-blind study. Epilepsia. 2017;58(10):1728-33.
42. COOKE PM, SNIDER RS. Some cerebellar influences on electrically-induced cerebral seizures. Epilepsia. 1955;4(1):19-28.
43. Velasco F, Carrillo-Ruiz JD, Brito F, Velasco M, Velasco AL, Marquez I, et al. Double-blind, randomized controlled pilot study of bilateral cerebellar stimulation for treatment of intractable motor seizures. Epilepsia. 2005;46(7):1071-81.
44. Benabid AL, Minotti L, Koudsié A, De Saint Martin A, Hirsch E. Antiepileptic effect of high-frequency stimulation of the subthalamic nucleus (corpus luysi) in a case of medically intractable epilepsy caused by focal dysplasia: A 30-month follow-up: Technical case report. Neurosurgery. 2002;50(6):1385-91.
45. Yang AI, Isbaine F, Alwaki A, Gross RE. Multitarget deep brain stimulation for epilepsy. J Neurosurg. 2023;140(1):210-7.
46. Skarpaas TL, Jarosiewicz B, Morrell MJ. Brain-responsive neurostimulation for epilepsy (RNS® System). Epilepsy Res. 2019;153:68-70.

47. Bergey GK, Morrell MJ, Mizrahi EM, Goldman A, King-Stephens D, Nair D, et al. Long-term treatment with responsive brain stimulation in adults with refractory partial seizures. Neurology. 2015;84(8):810-7.
48. Morrell MJ; RNS System in Epilepsy Study Group. Responsive cortical stimulation for the treatment of medically intractable partial epilepsy. Neurology. 2011;77(13):1295-304.
49. Heck CN, King-Stephens D, Massey AD, Nair DR, Jobst BC, Barkley GL, et al. Two-year seizure reduction in adults with medically intractable partial onset epilepsy treated with responsive neurostimulation: Final results of the RNS System Pivotal trial. Epilepsia. 2014;55(3):432-41.
50. Devinsky O, Friedman D, Duckrow RB, Fountain NB, Gwinn RP, Leiphart JW, et al. Sudden unexpected death in epilepsy in patients treated with brain-responsive neurostimulation. Epilepsia. 2018;59(3):555-61.
51. DiLorenzo DJ, Mangubat EZ, Rossi MA, Byrne RW. Chronic unlimited recording electrocorticography-guided resective epilepsy surgery: Technology-enabled enhanced fidelity in seizure focus localization with improved surgical efficacy. J Neurosurg. 2014;120(6):1402-14.
52. Skarpaas TL, Tcheng TK, Morrell MJ. Clinical and electrocorticographic response to antiepileptic drugs in patients treated with responsive stimulation. Epilepsy Behav. 2018;83:192-200.

CHAPTER 9

Management of Refractory Status Epilepticus

Jayakumari Nandana, KY Manisha, Ashalatha Radhakrishnan

ABSTRACT

Refractory status epilepticus (RSE) is characterized by persistent seizures despite an adequate trial of first- and second-line antiseizure medications (ASMs), i.e., benzodiazepines, phenytoin/fosphenytoin, levetiracetam, and valproate. Super refractory status epilepticus (SRSE) is characterized by continuing seizures despite 24 hours of intravenous anesthetic agents, or by the recurrence of seizures upon reduction or discontinuation of the same. About 10–40% of patients with status epilepticus, fail to respond to first- or second-line ASMs, with a mortality rate of around 40%. The crucial decision at this stage is whether to immediately initiate anesthetic medications or continue administering additional doses of alternative second-line medications. The Neurocritical Care Society recommends anesthetic medications for the treatment of RSE. Due to the absence of randomized clinical trials, the current management of RSE largely depends on retrospective data. Early appropriate and aggressive therapy is crucial for better outcomes in these patients.

Keywords: Refractory status epilepticus, Anesthetic agents, Immunomodulatory therapy, Outcome.

■ INTRODUCTION

Status epilepticus (SE) is considered a continuum of seizure activity that is classified based on its response to treatment, the management of which is one of the most challenging areas in neurocritical care, especially in a situation, where it becomes refractory to established protocols of management. The clinical staging and classification of SE helps in prognostication based on etiology and explores new therapeutic options, in addition to instilling a sense of urgency and diligence in the implementation of protocols.

■ DEFINITION

International League Against Epilepsy (ILAE) Task Force has proposed a definition for SE, which provides a framework for clinical diagnosis, investigation, and therapeutic approaches for each patient as well as aids in clinical and epidemiological studies.[1] The proposed definition of SE is as follows:[1] Status epilepticus is a condition resulting either from the failure of the mechanisms responsible for seizure termination or from the initiation of mechanisms that lead to abnormally, prolonged seizures (after time point t1). It is a condition that can have long-term consequences (after time point t2), including neuronal death, neuronal injury, and alteration of neuronal networks, depending on the type and duration of seizures.[1]

Treatment of SE commences with benzodiazepine administration (*stage 1:* early SE) followed by intravenous (IV) antiseizure medications (ASMs) such as phenytoin, fosphenytoin, levetiracetam or valproic acid (*stage 2:* established SE). SE becomes refractory when seizures continue (with definitions varying between 60–120 minutes across studies) despite initial first- and second-line therapies, and typically, this stage requires treatment with anesthetic agents [*stage 3:* refractory status epilepticus (RSE)].[2] Super refractory SE (SRSE) occurs when SE persists even after 24 hours of general anesthesia or reappears when the anesthetic agent is reduced or withdrawn.[3]

■ WHY IS IT IMPORTANT TO DEFINE REFRACTORINESS?

After refractoriness in SE is established, initiating a patient on IV anesthesia requires careful consideration of the therapy's potential to reverse seizure-induced neuronal damage, apoptosis, and inflammation, as well as any potential effects on pulmonary, gastrointestinal, and cardiorespiratory systems, requiring close observation in critical care units.[3] However, it is widely recognized that a prolonged period—weeks or even months—in a barbiturate or anesthetic coma for SRSE does not necessarily indicate a subpar functional outcome.[4] In addition to the age, history of prior seizures, seizure type, and extent of consciousness impairment, which are the core components of the Status Epilepticus Severity Score (STESS),[5] RSE duration and systemic complications like sepsis also have an impact on the outcome.[6] This highlights the urgency of developing novel therapeutic seizure termination and neuroprotective strategies once SRSE is established.

■ EPIDEMIOLOGY AND PROGNOSIS

The prevalence of RSE varies between 12 to 43% of cases with SE.[4,7-11] RSE does not respect age, gender, or ethnicity. The majority of patients present with generalized convulsive status, and after anesthetic drugs are administered, 40% of them develop into nonconvulsive or mild SE.[12] According to the literature, approximately 15% of adults have SRSE.[3,4,7-10] Patients with preexisting epilepsy account for between 34 to 60% of RSE episodes, albeit this number is probably impacted by referral bias and epidemiological trends.[12,13] The literature unequivocally indicates that outcomes of patients with RSE are closely related to its cause. While the etiology may be evident from the narrative in certain situations (such as severe traumatic brain injury, recent changes in ASMs, or recent neurosurgery), or in those without obvious cause, the blood collected for serum toxicology, autoimmune panel, alcohol, antiseizure medications (ASMs), and electrolyte levels may aid in etiological workup.[4,8,9] All patients with RSE require neuroimaging, even if a prior lesion is known, as an additional lesion or modification to an existing lesion may have triggered RSE.[9] In SRSE, our study identified separate treatment and electrophysiological prognostic variables.[9] The duration of the ICU stay, electroencephalogram (EEG) findings such as nonconvulsive SE in coma, spontaneous burst suppression, postictal diffuse attenuation, delay in starting anesthesia, and delay in initiating immunotherapy in new-onset refractory status epilepticus (NORSE) due to autoimmune encephalitis were independent predictors identified for poor outcome.[9] More than one-third of cases can be successfully treated with early commencement of treatment, strict management of these factors, especially in younger age groups, continuous EEG monitoring, and a comprehensive etiological workup.

CLINICAL PRESENTATIONS

The diagnosis of RSE is based on the fact that generalized convulsive SE persists after first- and second-line ASMs have been administered, and patients receiving treatment for generalized tonic–clonic or focal SE who do not regain consciousness after what is considered a sufficient "postictal" period should also be suspected of having RSE. Determining an appropriate postictal period in the absence of an EEG is challenging because it varies based on the type and duration of the seizure, the amount of AED used, and the etiology.

Refractory status epilepticus generally fits into one of the following categories at presentation: (1) Focal seizures with impaired awareness or generalized convulsive seizures and (2) stupor or coma after severe brain injury or following focal seizures with impaired awareness or generalized convulsive seizures.[13] In the hospital, the following circumstances call for an urgent EEG:[13] (1) Patients who remain unresponsive for 30 minutes or more after treatment for a focal SE with impaired awareness or generalized tonic–clonic seizure; (2) if a patient is found to be comatose without an alternate explanation following an emergency diagnostic workup; (3) In any patient who remains poorly responsive in conditions associated with epileptogenesis, such as brain surgery, particularly surgery performed after traumatic brain injuries, or tumor resection.

INSIGHTS INTO PATHOPHYSIOLOGY AND MANAGEMENT

In general, anesthetics agents and constant EEG monitoring are necessary to manage RSE.[14] The current recommendations suggest an early, sequential intervention, with benzodiazepines serving as the initial monotherapy and second-line medications being added one after the other if SE persists.[15] Gamma-aminobutyric acid type A (GABA-A) receptors are internalized following prolonged seizures in experimental models, but the concentration of glutamate receptors—especially N-methyl-D-aspartate (NMDA) receptors—increases at the synapse.[16] Moreover, GABA receptors experience reconfiguration upon internalization, thereby rendering them resistant to benzodiazepines. These receptors are also selectively shifted to extrasynaptic locations. These modifications include adjustments to the transmembrane gradient for chloride and the activity of GABA-A receptors, both of which reduce the ability of benzodiazepines to elevate inhibitory synaptic transmission.[17] Therefore, other mechanisms, such as changes in sodium ion channels or cholinergic mechanisms, may potentially be able to lessen the resistance to benzodiazepines.[16] Moreover, the intriguing options among the therapeutically available drugs are those that target NMDA receptors such as ketamine and, which target the α-amino-3-hydroxy-5-methyl-4-isoxazolepropionic acid receptor (also known as AMPA) receptor such as perampanel. Also involved in the breakdown of GABA-A receptor-mediated inhibition, these receptors seem to be overexpressed in SE. Promising outcomes have been obtained from studies examining the early administration of ketamine in animal models to treat RSE, frequently alongside other medications.[15] Furthermore, even when given following the onset of SE, ketamine's exceptional neuroprotective effects—achieved through the blockade of NMDA receptors—have been demonstrated by recent studies.[18]

MANAGEMENT STRATEGIES FOR REFRACTORY STATUS EPILEPTICUS

For the treatment of convulsive status epilepticus (CSE) in patients of all ages, from infants to adults, the American Epilepsy Society has laid up integrated treatment protocol and practical conclusions.[19] Based on the literature, the Neurocritical Care Society has also developed guidelines for CSE.[20] However, there is no consensus on how aggressively to treat nonconvulsive SE (NCSE) during RSE treatment.[21]

■ WHEN TO CONSIDER ANESTHETIC MEDICATIONS?

For patients with RSE, the Neurocritical Care Society recommends using anesthetic drugs.[20] Pentobarbital, propofol, and midazolam are the available continuous intravenous anesthetic alternatives for treating RSE or SRSE.[22] In addition, ketamine has been investigated as a potential substitute agent in recent reports. Nevertheless, in the absence of randomized controlled trials to offer recommendations on anesthetic medication selection for RSE treatment, management is largely dependent on retrospective data. Therefore, it is presently unknown which anesthetic third-line treatment for RSE provides better results, minimizes side effects, and is more effective in controlling seizures in the intensive care unit. It is very difficult to make meaningful comparisons between patients in most of the studies since they did not use standard data-gathering techniques.[22]

■ ANESTHETIC AGENTS

The selection of anesthesia is mostly influenced by the benefits and drawbacks, as well as the loading and maintenance doses of each drug, which are compiled in **Table 1**. The main objective of treating RSE with anesthesia is seizure control. However, in the management of SE, it is still unknown to what extent seizure suppression is optimal and whether burst suppression is needed. Additionally, there is debate on the length of time that should be spent in a therapeutic coma, even though a continuous infusion is normally maintained for 24-48 hours before weaning.[23] According to a recent observational study, there may be a correlation between a shorter and deeper therapeutic coma and a lower risk of complications from extended hospital stay as well as withdrawal seizures.[24] Hence, one should try to wean the patient off the anesthetics as soon as feasible after 24-48 hours with adequate seizure suppression. Other nonanesthetic AEDs ought to be added as well to prevent seizure recurrence.

As an NMDA receptor antagonist, ketamine is gaining importance as the most promising alternative among anesthetic medications for managing RSE. The main and intriguing theoretical advantage of ketamine is its unique mechanism of action. Ketamine targets a different pathway by acting on the NMDA receptor, in contrast to conventional anesthetics that operate on GABA receptors.[21] This distinct quality creates new opportunities for RSE management.[25,26] Furthermore, ketamine's neuroprotective properties have been extensively studied, yielding a wealth of scientific evidence that highlights its potential benefits.[18] Moreover, ketamine exhibits lower respiratory and cardiovascular adverse effects in comparison to other anesthetic agents. On the contrary, ketamine has several adverse effects, such as hallucinations, and sympathetic adrenergic actions, which might result in raised intracranial pressure, tachycardia, and hypertension.[27]

Ketamine has been shown to be effective for RSE and SRSE in two recent studies. In a single-center retrospective study, 69 children were treated with ketamine for RSE, for 66 patients (96%) ketamine infusions were started at a dose of 1 mg/kg/h, and the continuous infusion doses ranged from 1 to 7 mg/kg/h.[28] The infusion of ketamine lasted a median of 85.7 hours. When

TABLE 1: Anesthetic medications used for the treatment of refractory status epilepticus.

Drug	Mechanism of action	Loading dose	Maintenance dose	Onset of action/half-life	Advantages	Disadvantages
Midazolam	GABA receptor inhibitory action is potentiated by increasing the frequency of chloride channel opening	0.2 mg/kg (can vary between 0.03–0.5 mg/kg), at a maximum rate of 4 mg/minute	0.1–0.4 mg/kg/hour, (0.02–1.2 mg/kg/hour)	1.5 minutes/ 1.8–6.4 hours	Strong antiepileptic action, rapidly enters brain tissue and has a powerful short duration of action, and pharmacokinetic properties suitable for prolonged infusion without accumulation	Development of rapid and acute tolerance (tachyphylaxis) and hence risk of seizure relapse. A potent respiratory depressant, hypotension, hepatic and renal impairment are the other issues
Barbiturates (thiopental/pentobarbital)	Potentiation of GABA receptors through lengthening the duration of chloride channel opening rather than its frequency	2–7 mg/kg (thiopental) or 5–15 mg/kg (pentobarbital)	0.5–5 mg/kg/hour	10–40 seconds/ 3–22 hours (thiopental); <60 seconds/ 15–50 hours (phenobarbital)	Strong antiepileptic action, relatively safe profile, lowering of body temperature, and its theoretical neuroprotective effects	Profound tendency of accumulation resulting in a long half-life and longer recovery time, metabolized in liver, drug–drug interactions, hypotension, cardiorespiratory depression, pharmacological tolerance, and the risk of pancreatic and hepatic dysfunction

Continued

Continued

Drug	Mechanism of action	Loading dose	Maintenance dose	Onset of action/ half-life	Advantages	Disadvantages
Propofol	Modulation of GABA receptors	1 mg/kg, repeat after 5 minutes until seizures stop (maximum loading 10 mg/kg)	1–10 mg/kg/hour	15–30 seconds/ 4–7 hours	Very rapid onset and recovery, safe to be used in porphyria, no major drug–drug interaction, and less propensity of accumulation compared to barbiturates	• Hypotension, cardiorespiratory depression, pain at the injection site, and drug-induced involuntary movements • *Propofol infusion syndrome (PRIS)*: Potentially toxic effects on mitochondria and cellular metabolic functions, characterized by metabolic acidosis, lactic acidosis, rhabdomyolysis, hyperkalemia, hyperlipidemia, bradycardia and cardiac dysfunction, and renal failure
Ketamine	Noncompetitive NMDA receptor antagonist	0.5–2 mg/kg	0.6–5 mg/kg/hour	<30 seconds/ 2.5 hours	Lack of hypotension and cardiorespiratory depression and potential neuroprotective action	Hypertension, cardiac arrhythmia, pulmonary edema, and raises the intracranial pressure

(GABA: gamma-aminobutyric acid; NMDA: N-methyl-D-aspartate)

ketamine was given as the first anesthetic, the seizure termination was significantly more successful than when midazolam was tried first and failed—additionally, the negative effects while in the hospital were thought to be minimal and controllable, suggesting that ketamine can be used to treat RSE in adults and children in a safe and effective way.[28] In the second study, 68 adult patients with SRSE treated with ketamine between 2009 and 2018 were enrolled.[29] The median length of the ketamine infusion was 2 days, and the average dose was 2.2 ± 1.8 mg/kg/h. The seizure burden was reduced by 50% in the first 24 hours after starting ketamine treatment, and in 63% of cases, there was a complete cessation of seizures. In this study, 11 patients received multimodal monitoring in the intensive care unit, and the administration of ketamine was associated with a stable mean arterial pressure, which eventually decreased the need for vasopressors. Furthermore, in both traumatic and nontraumatic brain injury cases, there were no appreciable effects on cerebral blood flow, cerebral perfusion pressure, or intracranial pressure.[29] Based on these findings, ketamine treatment is beneficial for RSE, with higher dosages showing better hemodynamics without raising intracranial pressure. These findings are similar to that of earlier case studies and series, which indicate that ketamine is a useful treatment choice for those with hemodynamically unstable RSE.[30]

Refractory status epilepticus and SRSE cases collected by global registries aid in the understanding of the management of these patients as well as the development of improved protocols to rationalize the therapy. In a global audit published in 2019, 776 cases of RSE needing continuous anesthesia were prospectively collected by the authors.[31] In contrast to high-income countries, the introduction of anesthesia was delayed in middle-income countries. When it came to the first anesthetic drug used, there were notable regional variations. Globally, midazolam was the most often used initial agent, in 56% of cases, followed by propofol used in 35%, while in Europe, propofol was favored over midazolam. The choice or order of anesthetic medications did not influence the outcome. The administration of a barbiturate anesthetic did not result in a worse outcome. Even in cases where the first anesthetic agent failed, a greater percentage of patients responded to subsequent anesthetic medication cycles. Nevertheless, the neurological outcomes deteriorated after prolonged periods of SE and anesthesia use. Approximately, 158 patients needed three or more different anesthetic trials. After the third anesthetic was tapered, 49% of patients had seizure control, and 20% had a favorable neurological outcome. Therefore, the key to managing RSE and SRSE is persistence. For these reasons, we think it is crucial to continue therapy even in patients who are initially uncontrollable, since the major factor influencing the outcome is etiology rather than the length of the anesthetic medication.

■ INHALATIONAL HALOGENATED ANESTHETICS

In SRSE, volatile inhalational anesthetics, isoflurane and desflurane, have been investigated as an alternative salvage therapy. These anesthetics reduce seizure by enhancing GABA activity.[21] Benefits of inhalational anesthesia include a quick onset of effect and simple adjustment to EEG at the bedside. However, the literature available on inhalational anesthetics displays differences in treatment regimens, disparities in outcomes, and a lack of comparative groups. Additionally, the possibility of major side effects such as severe hypotension requiring vasopressors, atelectasis, and paralytic ileus, especially after prolonged use, limits the use of these anesthetics.[32]

ROLE OF CONTINUOUS EEG MONITORING

The majority of experts opine that continuous EEG monitoring (cEEG) is required while managing patients with RSE while on anesthetic medicines, even though there are no clear standards for the duration and EEG endpoint. Not only can cEEG monitoring aid in the diagnosis of NCSE but it can also be used to titrate anesthetic doses. Overuse of these potentially lethal medications can be harmful. Further research is required to clarify the optimal application of cEEG and its role in managing NCSE.

To evaluate the degree of anesthesia (burst-suppression pattern/suppression of varying degrees) and the cessation of ictal discharges during drug withdrawal, cEEG monitoring is recommended. The endpoint of EEG, i.e., whether to achieve total cessation of electrographic discharges versus burst-suppression pattern, is still debatable while handling a case with NCSE. Experts generally recommend that the most severe type of EEG suppression pattern, i.e., complete electrocerebral silence is linked to serious hemodynamic impairment. As a result, the goal is to attain burst suppression or eliminate ictal discharges. If cEEG facilities are not accessible, intermittent EEGs should be performed multiple times every 24 hours (the number and protocol are unknown as this is an optional practice that has not been validated), to titrate the medications.

CHOICE OF ANESTHETIC MEDICATION

Initially, one of the three traditional anesthetic medications should be administered; the choice will depend on the individual circumstances and preferences. Propofol infusions, however, have to be limited to 48 hours in cases where the benefits outweigh the risk. Propofol infusion syndrome is lethal, hence should be anticipated and cautious observation is necessary. In situations when alternative anesthetics fail or when drug-induced hypotension becomes a serious issue, ketamine should be taken into consideration. It is widely acknowledged that most physicians initiate patients with midazolam and switch to barbiturate anesthesia if it fails.

LEVEL OF ANESTHESIA REQUIRED

Anesthesia is often maintained to the level of burst suppression. Usually, all electrographic seizure activity terminates at this point. In other circumstances, milder anesthetic may also suppress activity. It is unclear if burst suppression is always necessary, and the available information is contradictory. Although seizures can be adequately controlled with burst suppression levels of anesthesia, there is a considerable risk of hypotension and other systemic consequences. Currently, it is the standard procedure to aim for burst suppression initially, then reduce the amount of anesthetic with prolonged episodes.

CYCLING AND DURATION OF ANESTHETIC CYCLES

It is customary to reverse anesthesia initially every 24–48 hours, and then reestablish it if seizures recur. Individual cycles get longer over time, and after a few weeks, anesthesia is frequently maintained for 5 days before attempts are made to reverse it.

SPEED OF WEANING OF ANESTHETICS

The recommended duration of use for these drugs is not yet clear. It is still feasible that in very prolonged SE, the hazards associated with anesthesia exceed those of SE, hence attempts should be made to withdraw anesthesia for longer periods. Sometimes seizures that recur after anesthesia withdrawal spontaneously subside. However, it is currently standard procedure for continuing anesthesia (with the previously indicated cycles of withdrawal and reinstitution). It is unclear how quickly anesthetics can be discontinued, however, trials that have tried rapid weaning have shown significant rates of recurrence and rebound seizures as a potential risk. Weaning it gradually over a few days seems appropriate.

■ ALTERNATIVE THERAPIES IN MANAGEMENT OF REFRACTORY STATUS EPILEPTICUS AND SUPER REFRACTORY STATUS EPILEPTICUS

Role of Immunomodulation in Super Refractory Status Epilepticus

Immunotherapy is indicated in RSE in two conditions: (1) Possible autoimmune encephalitis, either formally diagnosed or suspected leading to SE and (2) role of inflammation in epileptogenesis, and especially the activation of specific inflammatory signaling pathways such as the interleukin-1 receptor/toll-like receptor (IL-1R/TLR) pathway, both experimentally and in human tissue.[33] Many cryptogenic cases might be due to occult immunological diseases with antibodies that have yet to be identified, or due to the persistence of the SE that is in part at least due to immunological processes. Steroids may have additional nonimmunological effects, including the reversal of blood–brain barrier opening, which has a crucial influence on the persistence of seizure activity and which may reverse GABAergic inhibition and also effects intracranial pressure.[34,35] There is also evidence that suggests early immunotherapy may be beneficial even when a definite immune etiology is not identified.[36]

Patients are usually treated with first-line therapies: IV methylprednisolone (IVMP; 1 g per day for 5 days) combined with or followed by IV immunoglobulin (IVIG) (0.4 g/kg/d for five daily doses), and/or plasma exchange (five to seven sessions in total, every other day). These may be followed by second-line therapies: Rituximab, cyclophosphamide, mycophenolate, and azathioprine. In addition, there are newer alternative therapies in small case series or case reports that have been reported as effective including anakinra, bortezomib or tocilizumab.[37] These may be worth considering if dealing with treatment-resistant autoimmune epilepsy-related RSE/cryptogenic NORSE.

Repetitive Transcranial Magnetic Stimulation

Over time, there has been a growing body of evidence supporting the use of repetitive transcranial magnetic stimulation (rTMS) for medically-resistant epilepsy.[38] The noninvasive method has acquired significant appeal recently because of its ease of administration and relative safety. It has been used occasionally; however, the results have been inconsistent and varied. Similar to focal electroconvulsive treatment (ECT), small intracranial electrical currents that cause long-term depression and suppression of cortical excitability may be set up during low frequency (<1 HzrTMS). Eight children who had rTMS for SE/RSE were among the 21 patients in 11 studies in a systematic review.[39] The average length of treatment before using rTMS was 22 days, and the mean number of ASMs tried before rTMS was 7.5. There was a great deal of variation in the stimulation technique, frequency of stimulation, and length of therapy. Different regimens were given on different days. The response rate was good overall, ranging from 80–100%. However, it was not sustained, with 73.3% of the initial respondents experiencing a recurrence. The one benefit of rTMS is that it has a relatively safe profile and does not involve sedation, muscle relaxation, or medication modification. This analysis found that only one patient experienced temporary sensory problems in their leg, despite its potential to cause headaches, dizziness, and seizures (particularly during high-frequency stimulation). Recent case reports have investigated the potential usefulness of rTMS as a therapy for refractory epilepsia partialis continua in adults and children.[40,41]

Electroconvulsive Therapy

Among psychiatrists, electroconvulsive therapy (ECT) has long been an efficacious and well-established treatment for disorders including catatonia and refractory depression. It involves applying an electrical stimulus to set off a controlled generalized tonic–clonic seizure that produces the desired reaction through a process that has not yet been fully understood. When all other therapies fail, ECT has been used as a salvage therapy for SRSE based on the hypothesis that it increases seizure threshold. 19 patients with RSE got ECT, according to 14 original studies found in a systematic review.[42] The frequency of ECT therapy sessions varied greatly between the studies; one session per day was the most often reported frequency. The typical ECT treatment plan included daily sessions that lasted roughly 1 week. Of the 19 patients in this review, 11 (57.9%) had seizure reduction with the application of ECT and 7 (36.8%) had complete resolution and the best response was seen for NORSE and focal RSE. The length of time that ECT therapy produced a response ranged from 2 days to 8 years. The most common duration of time for ECT seizure control was 2 weeks to 3 months.

Emergency Surgery

When a patient has well-defined lesional epilepsy with consistent clinical, radiological, and electrophysiological data that contributes to RSE, neurosurgery may be a viable option. According to the review by Shorvon[14] and short case series,[43] emergency surgery appears to have a positive outcome with seizure freedom in a subset of patients. Numerous surgical methods have been performed, such as corpus callosotomy, multiple subpial transection, anatomic and functional hemispherectomy, lobar and multilobar resection, and localized cortical resection. The results were best for children and young people with cortical development abnormalities. As for the timing of the procedure, some cases underwent surgery as soon as 8 days after the onset of SE;[44] however, this should generally be taken into consideration based on the lesion's resectability and the patient's overall health, as surgery in and of itself shouldn't increase morbidity or mortality. Some experts, however, believe that surgery should be considered early in the course, after 2 weeks, as the evidence that is now available shows that late surgical treatment—that is, treatment performed after more than 30 days—has not produced the desired results, primarily because of the increasing morbidity brought on by extended hospital stays.[14]

Ketogenic Diet

One of the first treatment modalities for refractory seizures, the ketogenic diet (KD) is considered as a treatment option, particularly in the pediatric age group. It consists of two variations: The classic KD (4:1 fat to carbohydrate) or the modified Atkins diet (2:1), which induces ketosis and is thought to work by increasing GABA levels for purported anti-inflammatory effects. A retrospective case review conducted by Thakur et al. in adults with SRSE found that 90% of patients were able to achieve ketosis, and that the seizures stopped after a median of 3 days.[45] The side effects were mild; two patients experienced hypertriglyceridemia, and one patient experienced transient acidosis, which resolved without interrupting dietary treatment. About 270 adult SRSE patients on a KD showed an overall compliance of 45% and a combined effectiveness rate of 42% in a meta-analysis of 12 studies.[46] The patient can transition to a modified Atkins diet after their seizures are controlled. However, the main obstacle is the unpalatability, which leads to low adherence to these preparations. It is important to note that before starting KD, bowel mobility needs to be verified and the risk of sepsis needs to be ruled out. Careful blood glucose monitoring is recommended to avoid complications such as hypoglycemia.

Hypothermia

Both experimental and clinical research have demonstrated the therapeutic benefit of hypothermia in cases of cerebral hypoxia, and this use appears to be expanding. The mechanism appears to be multifaceted, encompassing reductions in intracellular acidosis, cellular apoptosis, free radical damage, and neuroinflammatory cascade. Although the potential role as an antiepileptic and anticonvulsant has been observed previously in vivo and in vitro studies, in the review by Motamedi on the use of therapeutic brain hypothermia and its prospects as a treatment for epilepsy, there was only limited data suggesting an antiepileptogenic effect.[47] The clinical evidence for SRSE is less robust, making it difficult to determine with certainty whether the anesthetic drug or hypothermia was the cause of the benefit.

The modest advantage appears to be only temporary, and seizures frequently return after reaching normothermia. The easiest methods of inducing hypothermia are direct application or gradual, cold saline infusion with rectal temperature monitoring. Clinical usage of hypothermia would probably require an implanted cooling device, which could make its application more difficult. However, even minor hypothermia might have adverse consequences; cardiac arrhythmias, coagulation abnormalities, immunosuppression, possibility of infection, thrombosis, and paralytic ileus are among them.[47] It is suggested that when combined with other anesthetics, the induction of mild therapeutic hypothermia (32–36°C) for a duration of 24–48 hours may represent a desperate option for SRSE. It is necessary to keep a close watch on the gastrointestinal, coagulation, and cardiac parameters given the considerable adverse effect profile. Additionally, as thiopentone can raise the risk of paralytic ileus in certain patients, it is best to avoid using it in combination.[47]

Magnesium

The inhibition of NMDA receptors by magnesium may be responsible for its antiepileptic properties. Its predominant function has been in the well-established conditions of preeclampsia and eclampsia. Zeiler's systematic review found that 50% of patients had seizure reduction or control; however, the effect was short-lived, as recurrences occurred when medication was stopped.[48] Across various studies, the continuous infusion ranged from 0.75 to 6 g/hour, after an IV loading that varied in dose from 3 to 6 g. To maintain a serum level of 3.5 mEq/L, a feasible regimen would be 1 g/hour infusion after 4 g IV loading over 20 minutes.[49] Despite the wide range of possible side effects, such as respiratory arrest, heart block, neuromuscular paralysis, etc., no substantial adverse effect was observed in the systematic review.[48] A urine output of more than 25 mL per hour with careful vital sign monitoring would be required. It is not yet recommended to routinely utilize magnesium infusion in noneclamptic seizures due to a lack of sufficient data.

Pyridoxine

The entity of pyridoxine-dependent epilepsy presenting with RSE has been well characterized, particularly in children. Diagnostic markers include elevated levels of cerebrospinal fluid (CSF) and plasma pipecolic acid and urine, as well as plasma α-aminoadipic semialdehyde (α-AASA).[50] The disease is characterized by a remarkable response to IV pyridoxine, with immediate cessation of clinical and electrographic seizures. Therefore, it is advised that a trial of IV or oral pyridoxine of 100 mg/day (up to a maximum of 500 mg/day) and continued at 30 mg/day in divided doses may be given routinely in SRSE, especially in children. Children who receive IV pyridoxine may experience hypotension, bradycardia, and apnea despite the very low adverse effect rate, particularly if they additionally are on other ASMs. Its effectiveness in adults is debatable, but considering the prevalence of acquired pyridoxine deficiency, particularly during pregnancy, its use is not unreasonable. Pyridoxine may be considered in patients with RSE.

■ NEW-ONSET REFRACTORY STATUS EPILEPTICUS

Episodes of RSE that develop as de novo NORSE are typically acute symptomatic in etiology, i.e., the result of an acute brain injury or drug intoxication or withdrawal. The most common types of acute brain injury presenting as NORSE include central nervous system infection, autoimmune encephalitis, brain tumor, traumatic brain injury, intracranial hemorrhage, and ischemic stroke.[13] Febrile infection-related epilepsy syndrome (FIRES), is considered a subcategory of NORSE rather than as a separate entity, as suggested earlier.[51]

As per recent international consensus recommendations, the treatment of NORSE with ASMs and anesthetic drugs during the initial 48 hours should be similar to acute treatment of RSE in other conditions.[52] They recommend that in contrast to RSE, in NORSE/FIRES, first-line immunotherapy—which may include corticosteroids (CS), IVIG, or therapeutic plasma exchange (TPE)—should be initiated within the first 72 hours of onset of SE. The KD and second-line immunotherapies should be initiated within 1 week in noninfectious NORSE/FIRES with inadequate response to first-line immune treatment. Because current evidence does not clearly support the use of any specific second-line immunological treatment over others, the choice should be based on suspected etiology.[53] If a pathogenic antibody is identified or an autoimmune process highly suspected, rituximab treatment should be the preferred treatment in most cases. In cryptogenic NORSE/FIRES without clinical features of a specific autoimmune encephalitis syndrome, IL-1 receptor antagonists or IL-6 blockers should be strongly considered.

■ STATUS EPILEPTICUS IN PREGNANCY

Status epilepticus in pregnancy (SEP) carries high risk of fetal death as has been reported by Hillesmaa et al.;[54] with fetal death noted in 50% cases and maternal death in 30% cases. According to EURAP data, SE is seen in 1.8% of pregnancies.[55] Managing SE in pregnancy is all the more complicated given the increased clearance of ASM during pregnancy secondary to increased hepatic metabolism, renal clearance, and decreased protein binding. The management is largely influenced by two factors: (1) Etiology of SE and (2) duration of pregnancy.[56,57]

The group of SEP in women without a history of epilepsy (NOSEP) differs significantly from the group of women with epilepsy (WWE) with SEP in terms of cause, course, and prognosis. In NOSEP, SE is most often caused by entities like posterior reversible encephalopathy syndrome (PRES), reversible cerebral vasoconstriction syndrome (RCVS), eclampsia, and cortical venous thrombosis (CVT). $MgSO_4$ is the treatment of choice for eclampsia in pregnancy.[58,59] Other than in eclampsia, there are no established guidelines for management of pregnancy-related SE. Magnesium supplementation has been shown to raise seizure threshold in animal and human studies, but the etiological contribution of magnesium deficiency to the onset and maintenance of epilepsy, as well as the degree to which it impacts AED efficacy, remains poorly understood. If SE occurs or persists despite treatment of the underlying cause, it is managed as per SE treatment guidelines.

However, it is recommended to avoid valproate, especially in the 1st trimester. Levetiracetam is the most frequently used ASM for benzodiazepine-refractory SEP as per the current survey.[60] If SE occurs early during pregnancy or takes a refractory course endangering the life of the pregnant woman, medical termination or rapid induction of (premature) delivery needs to be considered in interdisciplinary collaboration with the obstetricians and neonatologists. Pregnancies between completed and 32 weeks' gestation should preferably be terminated following induction of lung maturity; and in above completed 32 weeks' gestation, rapid termination may be sought.[61]

■ CONCLUSION

Early intervention and cessation of seizures are critical in SE. However, to prevent mortality and complications following RSE, it is essential to rely on evidence-based treatments when initiating intensive management with general anesthesia and coma therapy. Currently, no randomized control trials or guidelines are available for its optimal management. Improving RSE outcomes requires tailored care based on each patient's unique characteristics and underlying condition.

REFERENCES

1. Trinka E, Cock H, Hesdorffer D, Rossetti AO, Scheffer IE, Shinnar S, et al. A definition and classification of status epilepticus: Report of the ILAE Task Force on classification of status epilepticus. Epilepsia. 2015;56(10):1515-23.
2. Menon R, Radhakrishnan A, Radhakrishnan K. Status epilepticus. J Assoc Physicians India. 2013;61(8 Suppl):58-63.
3. Shorvon S. Super-refractory status epilepticus: An approach to therapy in this difficult clinical situation. Epilepsia. 2011;52 (Suppl 8):53-6.
4. Kantanen AM, Reinikainen M, Parviainen I, Ruokonen E, Ala-Peijari M, Bäcklund T, et al. Incidence and mortality of super-refractory status epilepticus in adults. Epilepsy Behav. 2015;49:131-4.
5. Rossetti AO, Logroscino G, Milligan TA, Michaelides C, Ruffieux C, Bromfield EB. Status Epilepticus Severity Score (STESS): A tool to orient early treatment strategy. J Neurol. 2008;255(10):1561-6.
6. Madžar D, Geyer A, Knappe RU, Gollwitzer S, Kuramatsu JB, Gerner ST, et al. Association of seizure duration and outcome in refractory status epilepticus. J Neurol. 2016;263(3):485-91.
7. Tian L, Li Y, Xue X, Wu M, Liu F, Hao X, et al. Super-refractory status epilepticus in West China. Acta Neurol Scand. 2015;132(1):1-6.
8. Jayalakshmi S, Ruikar D, Vooturi S, Alladi S, Sahu S, Kaul S, et al. Determinants and predictors of outcome in super refractory status epilepticus: A developing country perspective. Epilepsy Res. 2014;108(9):1609-17.

9. Jose J, Keni RR, Hassan H, Menon R, Sukumaran S, Cherian A, et al. Predictors of outcome in super refractory status epilepticus. Epilepsy Behav. 2021;118:107929.
10. Delaj L, Novy J, Ryvlin P, Marchi NA, Rossetti AO. Refractory and super-refractory status epilepticus in adults: A 9-year cohort study. Acta Neurol Scand. 2017;135(1):92-9.
11. Hassan H, Rajiv KR, Menon R, Menon D, Nair M, Radhakrishnan A. An audit of the predictors of outcome in status epilepticus from a resource-poor country: A comparison with developed countries. Epileptic Disord. 2016;18(2):163-72.
12. Claassen J, Hirsch LJ, Emerson RG, Mayer SA. Treatment of refractory status epilepticus with pentobarbital, propofol, or midazolam: A systematic review. Epilepsia. 2002;43(2):146-53.
13. Hocker SE, Britton JW, Mandrekar JN, Wijdicks EFM, Rabinstein AA. Predictors of outcome in refractory status epilepticus. JAMA Neurol. 2013;70(1):72-7.
14. Shorvon S, Ferlisi M. The treatment of super-refractory status epilepticus: A critical review of available therapies and a clinical treatment protocol. Brain. 2011;134(10):2802-18.
15. Amengual-Gual M, Sánchez Fernández I, Wainwright MS. Novel drugs and early poly-pharmacotherapy in status epilepticus. Seizure. 2019;68:79-88.
16. Joshi S, Rajasekaran K, Hawk KM, Chester SJ, Goodkin HP. Status Epilepticus: Role for etiology in determining response to benzodiazepines. Ann Neurol. 2018;83(4):830-41.
17. Burman RJ, Rosch RE, Wilmshurst JM, Sen A, Ramantani G, Akerman CJ, et al. Why won't it stop? The dynamics of benzodiazepine resistance in status epilepticus. Nat Rev Neurol. 2022;18(7):428-41.
18. Fujikawa DG. Starting ketamine for neuroprotection earlier than its current use as an anaesthetic/antiepileptic drug late in refractory status epilepticus. Epilepsia. 2019;60(3):373-80.
19. Glauser T, Shinnar S, Gloss D, Alldredge B, Arya R, Bainbridge J, et al. Evidence-based Guideline: Treatment of Convulsive Status Epilepticus in Children and Adults: Report of the Guideline Committee of the American Epilepsy Society. Epilepsy Curr. 2016;16(1):48-61.
20. Brophy GM, Bell R, Claassen J, Alldredge B, Bleck TP, Glauser T, et al. Guidelines for the evaluation and management of status epilepticus. Neurocrit Care. 2012;17(1):3-23.
21. Shin JW. Management strategies for refractory status epilepticus. Neurocrit Care. 2023;16:59-68.
22. Minicucci F, Ferlisi M, Brigo F, Mecarelli O, Meletti S, Aguglia U, et al. Management of status epilepticus in adults. Position paper of the Italian League against Epilepsy. Epilepsy Behav. 2020;102:106675.
23. Trinka E, Leitinger M. Management of status epilepticus, refractory status epilepticus, and super-refractory status epilepticus. Continuum (Minneap Minn). 2022;28(2):559-602.
24. Muhlhofer WG, Layfield S, Lowenstein D, Lin CP, Johnson RD, Saini S, et al. Duration of therapeutic coma and outcome of refractory status epilepticus. Epilepsia. 2019;60(5):921-34.
25. Gaspard N, Foreman B, Judd LM, Brenton JN, Nathan BR, McCoy BM, et al. Intravenous ketamine for the treatment of refractory status epilepticus: A retrospective multicenter study. Epilepsia. 2013;54(8):1498-503.
26. Espinosa L, Gomez M, Zamora A, Molano-Franco D. Refractory and super-refractory status epilepticus and evidence for the use of ketamine: A scope review. J Neurocrit Care. 2023;16(1):1-9.
27. Groth CM, Droege CA, Connor KA, Kaukeinen K, Acquisto NM, Chui SHJ, et al. Multicenter retrospective review of ketamine use in the ICU. Crit Care Explor. 2022;4(2):e0633.
28. Jacobwitz M, Mulvihill C, Kaufman MC, Gonzalez AK, Resendiz K, MacDonald JM, et al. Ketamine for management of neonatal and pediatric refractory status epilepticus. Neurology. 2022;99(12):e1227-38.
29. Alkhachroum A, Der-Nigoghossian CA, Mathews E, Massad N, Letchinger R, Doyle K, et al. Ketamine to treat super-refractory status epilepticus. Neurology. 2020;95(16):e2286-94.
30. Choi JW, Shin JW. Early combination therapy of ketamine and midazolam in patients with refractory status epilepticus in hemodynamic unstable state. J Epilepsy Res. 2021;11(2):150-3.
31. Ferlisi M, Hocker S, Trinka E, Shorvon S; International Steering Committee of the StEp Audit. The anaesthetic drug treatment of refractory and super-refractory status epilepticus around the world: Results from a global audit. Epilepsy Behav. 2019;101(Pt B):106449.
32. Mirsattari SM, Sharpe MD, Young GB. Treatment of refractory status epilepticus with inhalational anesthetic agents isoflurane and desflurane. Arch Neurol. 2004;61(8):1254-9.

33. Vezzani A, Rüegg S. The pivotal role of immunity and inflammatory processes in epilepsy is increasingly recognized: introduction. Epilepsia. 2011;52(Suppl 3):1-4.
34. Vezzani A, Balosso S, Aronica E, Ravizza T. Basic mechanisms of status epilepticus due to infection and inflammation. Epilepsia. 2009;50(s12):56-7.
35. Verhelst H, Boon P, Buyse G, Ceulemans B, D'Hooghe M, Meirleir LD, et al. Steroids in intractable childhood epilepsy: Clinical experience and review of the literature. Seizure. 2005;S14(6):412-21.
36. Holzer FJ, Seeck M, Korff CM. Autoimmunity and inflammation in status epilepticus: From concepts to therapies. Expert Rev Neurother. 2014;14(10):1181-202.
37. Foiadelli T, Santangelo A, Costagliola G, Costa E, Scacciati M, Riva A, et al. Neuroinflammation and status epilepticus: A narrative review unraveling a complex interplay. Front Pediatr. 2023;11:1251914.
38. Lefaucheur JP, Aleman A, Baeken C, Benninger DH, Brunelin J, Di Lazzaro V, et al. Evidence-based guidelines on the therapeutic use of repetitive transcranial magnetic stimulation (rTMS): An update (2014-2018). Clin Neurophysiol. 2020;131(2):474-528.
39. Zeiler FA, Matuszczak M, Teitelbaum J, Gillman LM, Kazina CJ. Transcranial Magnetic Stimulation for Status Epilepticus. Epilepsy Res Treat. 2015;2015:678074.
40. Agac B, Sharma K, Amorim-Leite R, Cho T. A Case of super-refractory epilepsia partialis continua successfully treated with repetitive transcranial magnetic stimulation (2854). Neurology. 2021;96:2854.
41. Chang D, Singhal NS, Tarapore PE, Auguste KI. Repetitive transcranial magnetic stimulation (rTMS) as therapy in an infant with epilepsia partialis continua. Epilepsy Behav Rep. 2021;18:100511.
42. Zeiler FA, Matuszczak M, Teitelbaum J, Gillman LM, Kazina CJ. Electroconvulsive therapy for refractory status epilepticus: A systematic review. Seizure. 2016;35:23-32.
43. Cuello-Oderiz C, Aberastury M, Besocke AG, Sinner J, Comas-Guerrero B, Ciraolo CA, et al. Surgical treatment of focal symptomatic refractory status epilepticus with and without invasive EEG. Epilepsy Behav Case Rep. 2015;4:96-8.
44. Ng YT, Rekate HL, Prenger EC, Chung SS, Feiz-Erfan I, Wang NC, et al. Transcallosal resection of hypothalamic hamartoma for intractable epilepsy. Epilepsia. 2006;47(7):1192-202.
45. Thakur KT, Probasco JC, Hocker SE, Roehl K, Henry B, Kossoff EH, et al. Ketogenic diet for adults in super-refractory status epilepticus. Neurology. 2014;82(8):665-70.
46. Ye F, Li XJ, Jiang WL, Sun HB, Liu J. Efficacy of and patient compliance with a ketogenic diet in adults with intractable epilepsy: A meta-analysis. J Clin Neurol. 2015;11(1):26-31.
47. Motamedi GK, Lesser RP, Vicini S. Therapeutic brain hypothermia, its mechanisms of action, and its prospects as a treatment for epilepsy. Epilepsia. 2013;54(6):959-70.
48. Zeiler FA, Matuszczak M, Teitelbaum J, Gillman LM, Kazina CJ. Magnesium sulfate for non-eclamptic status epilepticus. Seizure. 2015;32:100-8.
49. Lowe SA, Bowyer L, Lust K, McMahon LP, Morton M, North RA, et al. SOMANZ guidelines for the management of hypertensive disorders of pregnancy 2014. Aust NZJ Obstet Gynaecol. 2015;55(5):e1-29.
50. Stockler S, Plecko B, Gospe SM Jr, Coulter-Mackie M, Connolly M, van Karnebeek C, et al. Pyridoxine dependent epilepsy and antiquitin deficiency: Clinical and molecular characteristics and recommendations for diagnosis, treatment and follow-up. Mol Genet Metab. 2011;104(1-2):48-60.
51. Körtvelyessy P, Lerche H, Weber Y. FIRES and NORSE are distinct entities. Epilepsia. 2012;53(7):1276.
52. Wickström R, Taraschenko O, Dilena R, Payne ET, Specchio N, Nabbout R, et al. International consensus recommendations for management of new onset refractory status epilepticus (NORSE) including febrile infection-related epilepsy syndrome (FIRES): Summary and clinical tools. Epilepsia. 2022;63(11):2827-39.
53. Cabrera Kang CM, Gaspard N, LaRoche SM, Foreman B. Survey of the diagnostic and therapeutic approach to new-onset refractory status epilepticus. Seizure. 2017;46:24-30.
54. Hiilesmaa VK, Bardy A, Teramo K. Obstetric outcome in women with epilepsy. Am J Obstet Gynecol. 1985;152(5):499-504.
55. EURAP Study Group. Seizure control and treatment in pregnancy: Observations from the EURAP Epilepsy Pregnancy Registry. Neurology. 2006;66(3):354-60.
56. Rajiv KR, Radhakrishnan A. Status epilepticus in pregnancy: Etiology, management, and clinical outcomes. Epilepsy Behav. 2017;76:114-9.

57. Rajiv KR, Radhakrishnan A. Status epilepticus in pregnancy – Can we frame a uniform treatment protocol? Epilepsy Behav. 2019;101:106376.
58. Rajiv KR, Menon RN, Sukumaran S, Cherian A, Thomas SV, Nair M, et al. Status epilepticus related to pregnancy: Devising a protocol for use in the intensive care unit. Neurol India. 2018;66(6):1629.
59. Magpie Trial Follow-up Study Collaborative Group. The Magpie Trial: A randomised trial comparing magnesium sulphate with placebo for pre-eclampsia. Outcome for women at 2 years. BJOG. 2007;114(3):300-9.
60. Swor D, Juneja P, Constantine C, Mann C, Rosenow F, LaRoche S. Management of status epilepticus in pregnancy: A clinician survey. Neurol Res Pract. 2024;6(1):3.
61. Rosenow F, Mann C. Status epilepticus in pregnancy. Epilepsy Behav. 2023;138:109034.

CHAPTER 10

Management of Functional Seizures

Jayanti Mani, Aparna Ramakrishnan

ABSTRACT

Functional seizures (FS) are paroxysmal episodes of altered movement, sensation, or experience that mimic epileptic seizures, but not associated with epileptiform discharges in the brain but which, instead, have a psychological basis. FS are relatively common, estimated at 5–10% of outpatients in epilepsy clinics and 30% of inpatients in epilepsy monitoring units. Approximately 70% of patients with FS have current or previous psychogenic disorder, and approximately 10% of patients with FS have coexistent epilepsy. The delay in the diagnosis of FS from first symptom manifestation is an average of 7–9 years. Early diagnosis of FS is associated with better outcomes. Video electroencephalogram monitoring (VEEG) remains the gold standard for the diagnosis of epilepsy and psychogenic nonepileptic seizures (PNES). The key step after confirming the diagnosis of psychogenic seizures (PS) consists of communication of the diagnosis. Empathy and nonjudgmental attitude are the overarching principles for effective treatment of FS. The mainstay for the treatment of FS is psychotherapy, with cognitive behavioral therapy (CBT) being the technique with maximum reported efficacy. Psychopharmacologic agents play a limited role mainly in the treatment of comorbid mood, anxiety, or psychotic disorders. Individualized pharmacological and psychotherapeutic treatment plans are recommended based on the psychiatric evaluations. Treatment should not target complete cessation of events but should aim to improve ability to function at work and school and to help engage in personal relationships. The neurologist plays a key role in the discontinuation of unnecessary antiseizure medications and to calibrate lifestyle issues related to work and driving.

Keywords: Functional seizures, Psychogenic non-epileptic seizures, Pseudoseizures, Management.

INTRODUCTION

Functional seizures (FS) are paroxysmal episodes of altered movement, sensation, or experience than mimic epileptic seizures (ES), but not associated with epileptiform discharges in the brain but which, instead, have a psychological basis. FS are categorized as a conversion disorder (functional neurological symptom disorder) [Diagnostic and Statistical Manual of Mental Disorders, Fifth Edition (DSM-5) classification] and considered to be an involuntary response to emotional, physical, or social distress. The misdiagnosis of FS as epileptic events can lead to potentially harmful increase in the dosage of antiseizure drugs (ASD) and erroneous labeling as refractory epilepsy. This is borne out by the fact that one out of four to five patients admitted to video electroencephalogram (VEEG) monitoring units with a diagnosis of drug refractory epilepsy are identified to have nonepileptic events, majority of these being psychogenic in origin.[1]

TERMINOLOGY

The most appropriate terminology for these events is still a matter of debate. The most widely used term in current scientific literature is psychogenic nonepileptic seizures or PNES. Other labels used in the past include pseudoseizures, hysterical seizures, psychogenic seizures (PS), and nonepileptic attacks. The term pseudoseizures is now considered pejorative; on the other hand, the term nonepileptic attack would be too broad and include nonpsychogenic and nonepileptic events such as syncope and migraine. An argument could also be made against using the term "seizure" as this word in medical terminology implies an epileptic basis and thus "events" or "spells" may be more suitable. Recently, some researchers have proposed to refer to this condition as "dissociative seizures" or "functional seizures." Methods of communicating the PNES diagnosis to patients, produce different effects on their understanding, acceptance, and/or rejection.[3]

EPIDEMIOLOGY

Functional seizures are relatively common, estimated at 5-10% of outpatients in epilepsy clinics and 30% of inpatients in epilepsy monitoring units.[4] Prevalence estimates for FS range from 2 to 33/100,000,[5] but recently documented rates are much higher at 144/100,000.[6] FS occur across the age span but begin most commonly between the second and fourth decades of life.[7] Majority of patients are women in their reproductive years but the gender disparity is less obvious in the preadolescents, elderly, and the mentally challenged.[2] Academic failure, childhood abuse, and family history of epilepsy are frequently seen with a younger onset age[8] and medical comorbidities are more prevalent at a later age of onset.

MECHANISMS IN FUNCTIONAL SEIZURES

Although FS are considered a mental health condition, there is still little agreement on the psychological mechanisms underlying these events. As FS is a group of symptoms and not a disease or a syndrome, the underlying etiology is expected to be heterogeneous.[9] In FS, "patients who show difficulty in expressing conflicts verbally, sometimes express distress somatically."[10] FS with motor symptoms is mainly represented in the category of conversion (somatoform disorders). However, when symptoms affect consciousness, FS would be better represented within dissociative disorders. Dissociation is considered a defense mechanism that helps the individual in coping with traumatizing events. In that sense, FS often follow stressful or traumatic events that generate a dissociation of the mental organization. The recently proposed "integrative cognitive model" (Fig. 1) accommodates current research on experiential, psychological, and biological risk factors for the development of FS into one comprehensive hypothesis.[11] However, in view of the considerable heterogeneity of the medical context and the clinical presentations it is not certain that a single universal model can capture the full range of PNES and its mechanisms.

PSYCHIATRIC COMORBIDITY

Approximately 70% of patients with FS have current or previous psychogenic disorder. Functional or "medically unexplained" symptoms are found in 60-80% of patients.[7]

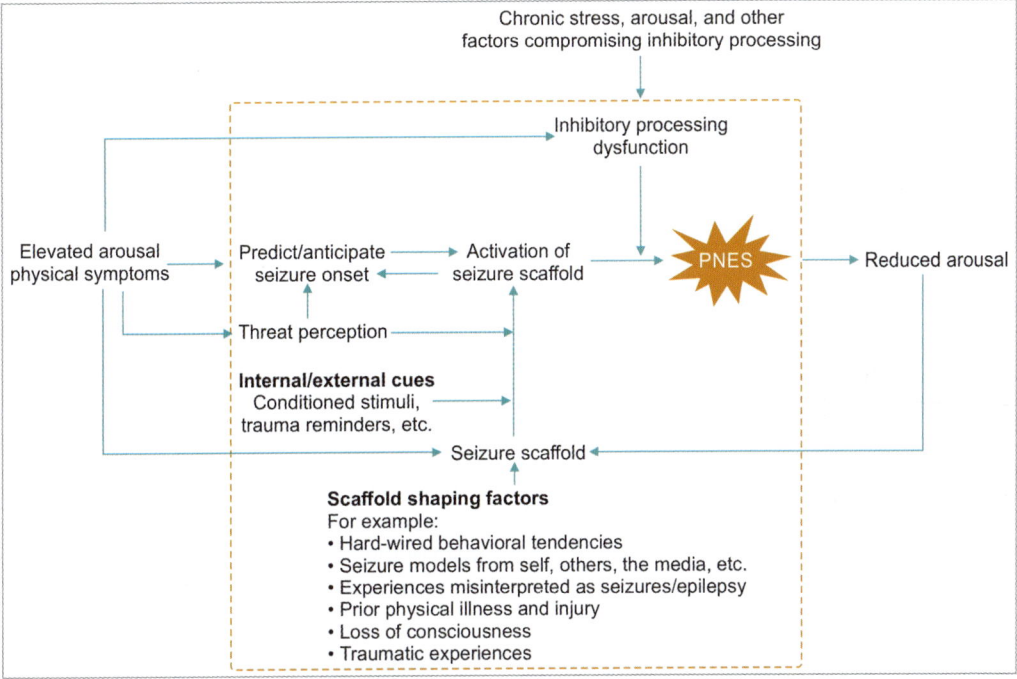

FIG. 1: Integrated cognitive model:[9] The figure hypothesizes on how rather than why psychogenic nonepileptic seizures (PNES) arise. Functional seizures are experiential and behavioral paroxysms due to activation of a learnt idea of a seizure, or "seizure scaffold." Essential components of the process are represented in the dashed area. Although abnormal arousal is frequently part of the functional seizures (FS) process, it is not an essential for FS generation. Strong activation of the seizure scaffold in the presence of an inhibitory processing dysfunction may be sufficient to trigger an attack even in the absence of heightened arousal. Recognized risk factors for FS such as a history of traumatization, emotional dysregulation, alexithymia, psychopathology, and heightened suggestibility will confer vulnerability to the processes depicted but are neither necessary nor sufficient in this account.

In a systematic review, psychiatric comorbidities had a prevalence of 53–100% in the FS groups, post-traumatic stress disorder (PTSD) and personality disorders were higher in the FS than in epilepsy.[12] Depression is the most prevalent comorbidity at 40%,[13] followed by anxiety 22–29%[14] and PTSD 30%.[15] FS and associated PTSD rates are even higher among war veterans at 58–64%.[16] Certain *personality disorders* like the borderline personality disorder or the cluster C personality (avoidant, dependent, or obsessive-compulsive) are also disproportionately high in some series of FS patients.[14,17] Children with PNES demonstrate lower rates of psychiatric comorbidities[8] including adjustment disorder (17%), somatic symptoms and related disorders (12%), neurodevelopmental disorders (11%), depression (6%), and anxiety (3%).

■ PSYCHOLOGICAL TRAUMA AND STRESSFUL LIFE EVENTS

Psychological trauma and previous life adversity play a significant role in the development of PNES, with 50–70% reporting antecedent trauma viz. increased rates of reported childhood abuse, sexual trauma in PNES patients.[18] Childhood trauma affects brain maturation especially in limbic and prefrontal areas, that leads to poor emotional regulation in relation to stress.[19] While mild stress may precipitate PNES in susceptible individuals, chronic or major psychological trauma may lead to PNES even in the absence of susceptibility.

Childhood Neglect and Family Dysfunction

A 2018 meta-analysis of stressors in persons with functional disorders corroborated that while a history of distressing life events was common, but maltreatment and neglect in childhood presented a bigger risk for FS than sexual or physical abuse.[20] In a series of patients with traumatic events, family dysfunction and bereavement were also present in two-thirds of cases, suggesting that family dysfunction and affective disorders, are the most common perpetuating factors of functional neurological disorders.[21]

Insecure Attachment Styles

Lack of reliable and nurturing figures to offer support in times of crisis, especially in childhood, leads to insecure attachment styles.[22] Maladaptive coping styles create a state of vulnerability to psychiatric disorders resulting in social anxiety and problems with interpersonal functioning. An episode can remove patients from interpersonally challenging situations and a ready escape mechanism is reinforced.[11] "Sick role" provides secondary reinforcement. Physician-related illness misattribution, delay in diagnosis, prescription of AEDs can be additive factors.

■ OTHER COMORBIDITIES

Approximately 10% of patients with FS have coexistent epilepsy[23] and in the cohort with intellectual disability the ratio of comorbid epilepsy is up to 30%.[23] Chronic pain, sleep issues, migraine, asthma, and history of head injury are also found more in patients with PNES than in the general population. Hence, it is difficult to establish whether a co-occurring condition is a true comorbidity, a predisposition, or an underlying cause of PNES.[24] Coexisting poorly defined (probably psychogenic) conditions such as "fibromyalgia" and unexplained "chronic pain" have a high predictive value of 70–80% for FS.[25]

Importantly, it is no longer necessary to identify an underlying psychological cause to make the diagnosis of PNES, as these factors may not become apparent until extensive psychotherapy is completed. In the DSM-5, the association of functional neurologic symptoms to a circumstantial trigger at the onset of the illness is no longer a requirement for the diagnosis.

■ MANAGEMENT OF FUNCTIONAL SEIZURES

The key components of effective management include:
- Establishing a diagnosis
- Communicating the diagnosis
- Evaluation for psychiatric comorbidity and its treatment
- Withdrawal of antiseizure medications (AEDs)

Establishing Diagnosis

The delay in the diagnosis of FS from symptom manifestation is reported to be an average of 7–9 years.[26] Clinical suspicion is key, and obtaining the description of the events is vital. However, it is equally important to look for other clues beyond the "seizure behavior", viz. the context in which the events occur and also other coexistent symptoms and illnesses. Mental status evaluation helps to identify psychological comorbidities in order to plan further treatment.

Clinical Evaluation

The interview: Obtaining details of seizure behavior will rely heavily on patient and eyewitness interviews. Events occur suddenly and accuracy of reporting by eyewitnesses can be variable. Moreover, both epileptic and nonepileptic events can have a wide range of behaviors, and hence mimic each other. A gentle and measured approach to the patient interview is helpful. Home videos captured on smart phones can prove to be an asset, but these may capture only part of the event.

Event Behavior

The patient often reveals a period of "headiness" or head pain lasting several minutes leading to the event. The patient also admits to being at least partially aware of the surroundings but being unable to respond.

Certain symptoms and event behaviors may strongly suggest FS **(Box 1)**. However, no single symptom can conclusively differentiate true epileptic events from FS. There may be value in considering clusters of features rather than a small number of single items.

As a rule of thumb, FS events last longer than ES and an episode lasting >10 minutes should raise the suspicion for FS.[27] ES exhibit a well-characterized onset, reach the peak of the clinical manifestations within a minute, and are followed, within a few minutes, by the ictal offset. On the other hand, PNES patients could be prolonged and have waxing and waning of symptoms with periods of inactivity.

Event Frequency and Triggers

Event frequency is higher in patients with FS than those with epilepsy. Recurrent hospital admissions with apparent seizure status or daily convulsive events suggest PNES[26] especially when reported by a well

> **BOX 1: Semiologic features that distinguish functional seizures from epileptic seizures.**
>
> - Signs that favor functional seizures:
>   - Long duration
>   - Fluctuating course
>   - Side-to-side head movements
>   - Pelvic thrusting and side-to-side movements
>   - Dystonic body posturing
>   - Closure of the eyes during event
>   - Ictal crying
>   - Memory recall of period when patient was "unconscious"
>   - Occurrence from "pseudosleep"
> - Signs that favor epileptic seizures:
>   - Occurrence from sleep
>   - Stertorous breathing
>   - Postictal confusion
> - Signs that are not discriminatory:
>   - Gradual onset
>   - Nonstereotyped events
>   - Tongue bite
>   - Urinary incontinence
>   - Opisthotonus
>   - Flailing or thrashing limbs
>
> *Source:* Adapted from Avbersek and Sisodiya JNNP, 2010.

and alert patient. Specific *event triggers* such as "stress" and "getting upset," pain, certain movements, sounds and lights; and the *circumstances* in which attacks occur, e.g., occurrence in the physician's office or waiting room or during the examination are typical features. Often FS could arise from periods of "pseudosleep", on the other had occurrence from documented EEG sleep has a 100% specificity for ES.[27,28]

Confirmation of Diagnosis

On suspicion of PNES, prompt referral to an epilepsy center is recommended, as early diagnosis of PNES is associated with better outcomes. Overinterpretation of the outpatient EEG is often the reason for

FS being misdiagnosed as epileptic in the early phase of diagnosis. This may be due to EEGs being reported by personnel without adequate training.

Video Electroencephalogram Monitoring

The VEEG remains the gold standard for the diagnosis of epilepsy and PNES and allows to establish the diagnosis with a high level of confidence and reliability.[29] Simultaneous recording of a normal EEG with the habitual paroxysmal event establishes the diagnosis of FS. This removes ambiguity and avoids having to revisit the diagnosis or arbitrary reintroduction of AEDs in breakthrough events. Hence, best-practice diagnosis should include VEEG for any individual with suspected FS.[30]

Induction of Seizures

Seizure-related provocative techniques exhibit good sensitivity and excellent specificity for inducing FS and help shorten the length of the hospitalization or VEEG required for the diagnosis.[31] A range of methods have been employed as triggers from simple verbal suggestions to a variety of placebos such as saline injections, perfumes, and olfactive stimulants, and vibrating tuning fork on the forehead as well as standard activation procedures employed in EEG such as hyperventilation and photic stimulations. Ethical concerns have been raised about the employment of some of the methods. The ethical issues may be circumvented by use of only the standard activation procedures that are routinely employed in EEG as these have been shown to exhibit diagnostic power similar to the induction maneuvers.

Limitations of Video Electroencephalogram in Diagnosis of Functional Seizures

The absence of epileptiform correlates during the habitual event is the basis for diagnosis of FS. However, some true ES may also not demonstrate epileptiform discharges on scalp EEG, e.g., simple partial seizures with only sensory or experiential auras, brief dialeptic events or very focal motor seizures, and excessive muscle activity due to muscle tightening or violent motor activity can obscure scalp EEG patterns, e.g., in hypermotor frontal lobe seizures. Hence, the absence of an ictal pattern must be interpreted with reference to the semiology on the video, and the whole clinical context should also be taken into consideration.

Serum Prolactin Levels

Doubling of serum prolactin (PRL) values 10-20 minutes after the onset of the ictus compared to preictal values helps discriminate generalized tonic clonic epilepsy from PNES.[32] False positives can occur with use of tricyclic antidepressants or antipsychotics and in syncope. PRL levels may also fail to rise in true ES from the frontal lobe. Hence, PRL levels, are not nearly as reliable as VEEG and only have a role when VEEG is not available.

Clinical Scoring Systems

More recently various scoring systems have been proposed to facilitate a diagnosis of FS,[33-35] many of these are promising but their complexity may hinder widespread use. The clinical functional seizure score[36] is a simpler score based on demographic and semiological factors, and psychiatric comorbidities. These scoring systems await validation but have potential to be part of clinical practice especially when access to epileptologists and VEEG units is limited.

Communicating the Diagnosis

The key step after confirming the diagnosis of PNES consists of communication of the diagnosis. This also serves as a therapeutic opportunity to provide psychoeducation about the nature of the disorder, reinforce engagement in treatment, and foster an effective interaction with the healthcare system. Various communication protocols have been proposed on how the diagnosis should be delivered[37] and these have been consolidated in **Table 1**. Empathy and nonjudgmental attitude are the overarching principles for effective treatment of FS, the diagnosis is to be communicated in a clear yet tactful and sympathetic nonjudgmental manner, and the condition should be identified with a name viz. nonepileptic attacks or FS. The right choice of words during the conversation is important, and terms like "hysterical" or "pseudoseizures" should be clearly avoided. Presence of family or loved ones when the diagnosis is conveyed, helps better understanding and acceptance of the condition. Maintaining a confident and yet supportive approach throughout the process of diagnosis and treatment is the cornerstone of successful management. For a subset of patients with PNES, awareness that their events are psychogenic may prove therapeutic in itself. On the other hand, the initial reactions of the patient and family to the diagnosis have a major influence on treatment outcomes.[38]

TABLE 1: Suggested communication protocols for diagnosis delivery.

Covered topic	Communication points delivered to patient
Negative diagnosis	• What you do not have? (i.e., epilepsy) • What you do not need? (i.e., treatment with antiepileptic drugs)—unless needed for other indications
Diagnostic method	• How the diagnosis was made (i.e., VEEG captured typical event) • "It is common!" frequently seen in long-term monitoring units
Genuine symptoms	Symptoms are real, not fabricated
Explanatory model (positive diagnosis)	Role of accumulating risk factors over time and automatic functional brain patterns
Suggestion	Some patients improve with reassurance that their events are not epileptic, once the diagnosis is explained
Treatment and expectations	• There are effective treatments • Psychotherapy works though skills learning, "brain retraining" • There is no sudden cure, treatment requires time and training

Source: La France, et al., Epilepsia 2013.

Evaluation and Management of Psychological Comorbidity

When FS are suspected by the neurologist, evaluation by a mental health professional before the diagnosis is confirmed can facilitate crafting an explanatory model for the psychogenic etiology of the event. Once the functional nature of seizures is established, a comprehensive psychiatric evaluation and psychometric testing is recommended in all FS. Predisposing, precipitating, and perpetuating factors must be investigated.

Neuropsychological Tests

Neuropsychological tests can help to isolate distinct cognitive, emotional, and personality features of PNES patients, but have limited value for the differential diagnosis with epilepsy. A variety of structured clinical interview methods and assessment scales may be used to assist in establishing the underlying comorbidities **(Table 2)**.

More recently suggested scoring systems to establish diagnosis of FS that await validation are discussed earlier.

Patients with PNES exhibited high scores in the domain of neuroticism, which are associated with "distress proneness and a

TABLE 2: Psychological assessment batteries to be used in evaluation of functional seizures (FS) patients.

Psychiatric interview techniques for evaluation	• Structured clinical interview for Diagnostic and Statistical Manual diagnosis (SCID) • Mini-international neuropsychiatric interview (MINI)
Assessment of personality factors	• Minnesota multiphasic personality inventory (MMPI) or the MMPI-2 • Millon clinical multiaxial inventory (MCMI)
Assessment of dissociation	• Dissociative seizure likelihood (probability) score (DSLS) • Multiscale dissociation inventory • Somatoform dissociation questionnaire • Dissociative experiences scale

persistent tendency to experience life events negatively and alexithymia traits that is correlated with a difficulty in recognizing and describing emotional states.[39]

Management of the Psychological Comorbidities

Compared to other psychiatric disorders, the evidence base for management of FS is limited.[40]

Psychological Therapies

Recent evidence suggests that psychological approaches are more effective. A 2017 meta-analysis of 13 studies found that 82% of persons with FS who completed a psychotherapy treatment protocol had a reduction in seizure frequency of 50% or more.[41]

Nearly all psychotherapy modalities include some form of psychoeducation and many offer similar or overlapping tools (e.g., grounding and distraction techniques, relaxation training, emotion recognition, and regulation skills training).

Cognitive behavioral therapy (CBT) currently exhibits the most robust experimental and clinical evidence of efficacy.[42] In a randomized clinical trial, patients who had CBT plus standardized medical therapy reported their FS as less bothersome, had a longer period of seizure freedom prior to follow-up, and reported better health-related quality of life, less impairment in psychosocial functioning, less overall psychologic distress, and fewer somatic symptoms compared to those who had medical treatment alone.[43]

Psychodynamic therapy can also be considered when FS are hypothesized to originate from dysfunctional early life relationships.

Prolonged exposure technique is a form of CBT used to treat comorbid PTSD.[44]

Interpersonal therapy is based on the hypothesis that FS stem from disturbed interpersonal relationships and aims to identify and change the dysfunctional relationship patterns.[45] *Family therapy* would be useful to target high levels of family dysfunction often identified. in FS patients.[46] *Mindfulness-based psychotherapy* is employed when FS originate from experiential avoidance.[47] Group therapy[48] and *hypnotherapy*[49] are other available strategies.

Psychopharmacologic Agents

Current evidence does not establish the additional value of pharmacological agents such as SSRIs over psychological treatments like CBT in management of FS.[50] However, psychopharmacologic agents should be considered for the treatment of identified comorbid mood, anxiety, or psychotic disorders, and possibly to treat somatoform symptoms. The choice of drug should be based on principles that guide treatment of the identified comorbidity.[37]

Individualized pharmacological and psychotherapeutic treatment plans are recommended based on the psychiatric evaluations.[51] Most of these therapies need to be continued for long periods. Patient participation and compliance can be a challenge impacting long-term outcomes.[52] Remaining flexible in terms of psychotherapeutic modality also allows treating clinicians to change strategies over time based on an individual's needs.

Once control is achieved, ongoing psychotherapy in the form of booster sessions is advisable, to reinforce learned strategies and maintain earlier gains. Focus should be to restore functioning at work, engaging in relationships and daily activities rather than on complete event freedom. This may need the adoption of other measures such as occupational therapy and vocational rehabilitation.

Discontinuation of Antiseizure Medications

Antiseizure medications have no role in the treatment of FS and can be a source of potential harm. The pharmacologic treatment of pure FS patients should commence with early tapering and discontinuation of AEDs. AEDs having a beneficial effect, i.e., use in comorbid mood disorders and migraine, e.g., valproate or lamotrigine should only be continued in lowest effective doses. In patients with mixed ES and PNES, the number and doses of the AEDs should be reduced to the minimum necessary. Abrupt discontinuation of AEDs should be strongly discouraged.

■ EPILEPSY AND FUNCTIONAL SEIZURES: "DUAL DIAGNOSIS"

About 10% of patients with FS PNES[53] also have true ES. The basis of the development of PNES in epilepsy patient include: (1) Psychiatric comorbidities correlated to epilepsy, (2) the presence of a "seizure scaffold" on which PNES ensues; and (3) the development of substitute symptoms (in particular in patients recovering from epilepsy) to obtain secondary gains such as caregiver attention, monetary compensation, or work avoidance. A dual diagnosis is harder to establish and manage than isolated PNES.

■ ROLE OF THE NEUROLOGIST: MULTIDISCIPLINARY TEAM APPROACH

Neurologists and mental health professionals should be part of the multidisciplinary team that presents the results of the diagnostic investigations and constructs the treatment plan. The neurologist plays a key role in the discontinuation of unnecessary AEDs and calibrate lifestyle issues related to work and driving. A customized plan should be devised to avoid unnecessary admissions, including how to communicate with emergency personnel. Utilization of medical services is likely to reduce after a VEEG established diagnosis of FS.[54] The neurologist would be required to address other comorbid medical conditions, viz., headaches or ES. The neurologist should also remain available in case new semiologies or symptoms arise.[55] Many persons with FS have a difficult time adhering to the diagnosis and the treatment recommendations.[56] At times a polarizing view of neurologists about FS as a purely psychological problem versus perception by the patients and families of FS at least partly as a physical problem may hinder effective communication and generate discordant treatment expectation.[57] Hence, close attention should be paid to communication patterns. The explanation of the diagnosis should not be seen as a one-time discussion, but rather as a process that may require multiple contacts with the individual and their family. Continued engagement with the neurologist facilitates the gradual acceptance of the diagnosis.

■ TREATMENT OUTCOMES

Long-term outcomes in FS are modest with 50–80% continuing to have events when last assessed.[58] Outcomes are more favorable with ongoing active intervention.[52] Comorbid epilepsy or psychiatric illness, younger onset age, and elaborate seizure semiology predict poor outcomes whereas earlier intervention, better acceptance of the condition, higher level of education and functioning, and good social support predict better outcomes.[59] Most studies have focused on event frequency as a measure of efficacy, but reduced episode length, retained awareness, or increased ability to recognize a prodrome and moving to a safe location would all be signs of therapeutic success. Treatment should aim to improve ability to function and remain engaged in personal relationships and work or school. Other treatment goals include overall improved mental health and reduced unnecessary medical utilization. At times, FS may abate only to be seemingly replaced by worsened anxiety or mood symptoms. Although, this may appear to be a step sideways, these psychiatric symptoms are often more actionable and a part of patients' journeys toward wellness.

■ CONCLUSION

Functional seizures or psychogenic non-epileptic seizures (PNES) are a type of seizure that look like epileptic seizures but are actually caused by psychological factors, such as stress or trauma, rather than abnormal electrical activity in the brain.

Misdiagnosis is common leading to overuse of antiepileptic drugs that contribute to a poor quality of life.

Clinical suspicion and video EEG monitoring are the ways to establish the diagnosis. Psychotherapy and withdrawal of antiepileptic medications are the two cornerstones of management of FS. The use of psychopharmacology is limited and restricted to the treatment of the identified psychiatric comorbidity. Results of psychotherapy are best if begun early in the course of the illness.

■ ACKNOWLEDGMENT

We sincerely appreciate the assistance provided by Dr S Kamatchi in the preparation of this manuscript.

REFERENCES

1. American Psychiatric Association. Diagnostic and Statistical Manual of Mental Disorders, 5th edition. Washington, DC: American Psychiatric Publishing; 2013.
2. Asadi-Pooya AA, Sperling MR. Epidemiology of psychogenic nonepileptic seizures. Epilepsy Behav. 2015;46:60-5.
3. Asadi-Pooya AA, Brigo F, Mildon B, Nicholson TR. Terminology for psychogenic non-epileptic seizures: Making the case for "functional seizures". Epilepsy Behav. 2020;104:106895.
4. Benbadis SR, O'Neill E, Tatum WO, Heriaud L. Outcome of prolonged video-EEG monitoring at a typical referral epilepsy center. Epilepsia. 2004;45(9):1150-3.
5. Benbadis SR, Hauser WA. An estimate of the prevalence of psychogenic non-epileptic seizures. Seizure. 2000;9(4):280-1.
6. Goleva SB, Lake AM, Torstenson ES, Haas KF, Davis LK. Epidemiology of functional seizures among adults treated at a university hospital. JAMA Netw Open. 2020;3(12):e2027920.
7. Reuber M. Psychogenic nonepileptic seizures: answers and questions. Epilepsy Behav. 2008;12(4):622-35.
8. Reilly C, Menlove L, Fenton V, Das KB. Psychogenic non epileptic seizures in children: A review. Epilepsia. 2013;54(10):1715-24.
9. Brown RJ, Reuber M. A Psychological and psychiatric aspects of psychogenic non-epileptic

seizures (PNES): A systematic review. Clin Psychol Rev. 2016;45:157-82.
10. Stone J, LaFrance WC Jr, Brown R, Spiegel D, Levenson JL, Sharpe M. Conversion disorder: current problems and potential solutions for DSM-5. J Psychosom Res. 2011;71(6):369-76.
11. Brown RJ, Reuber M. Towards an integrative theory of psychogenic non-epileptic seizures (PNES). Clin Psychol Rev. 2016;47:55-70.
12. Diprose W, Sundram F, Menkes DB. Psychiatric comorbidity in psychogenic nonepileptic seizures compared with epilepsy. Epilepsy Behav. 2016;56:123-30.
13. Walsh S, Levita L, Reuber M. Comorbid depression and associated factors in PNES versus epilepsy: Systematic review and meta-analysis. Seizure. 2018;60:44-56.
14. Bermeo-Ovalle A, Kanner AM. Comorbidities in psychogenic nonepileptic seizures. In: LaFrance Jr WC, Schachter SC (Eds). Gates and Rowan's nonepileptic seizures, 4th edition. Cambridge: Cambridge University Press; 2018. pp. 245-56.
15. Fiszman A, Alves-Leon SV, Nunes RG, D'Andrea I, Figueira I. Traumatic events and posttraumatic stress disorder in patients with psychogenic nonepileptic seizures: a critical review. Epilepsy Behav. 2004;5(6):818-25.
16. Salinsky M, Rutecki P, Parko K, Goy E, Storzbach D, O'Neil M, et al. Psychiatric comorbidity and traumatic brain injury attribution in patients with psychogenic nonepileptic or epileptic seizures: a multicenter study of US veterans. Epilepsia. 2018;59(10):1945-53.
17. Lacey C, Cook M, Salzberg M. The neurologist, psychogenic nonepileptic seizures, and borderline personality disorder. Epilepsy Behav. 2007;11(4):492-8.
18. Bowman ES. Posttraumatic stress disorder, abuse, and trauma. In: LaFrance Jr WC, Schachter SC (Eds). Gates and Rowan's nonepileptic seizures, 4th edition. Cambridge: Cambridge University Press; 2018. pp. 231-44.
19. Paquola C, Bennett MR, Lagopoulos J. Understanding heterogeneity in grey matter research of adults with childhood maltreatment -a meta-analysis and review. Neurosci Biobehav Rev. 2016;69:299-312.
20. Ludwig L, Pasman JA, Nicholson T, Aybek S, David AS, Tuck S, et al. Stressful life events and maltreatment in conversion (functional neurological) disorder: systematic review and meta-analysis of case-control studies. Lancet Psychiatry. 2018;5(4):307-20.
21. Reuber M, Howlett S, Khan A, Grünewald RA. Non-epileptic seizures and other functional neurological symptoms: predisposing, precipitating, and perpetuating factors. Psychosomatics. 2007;48(3):230-8.
22. Villagrán A, Lund C, Duncan R, Lossius MI. The effect of attachment style on long-term outcomes in psychogenic nonepileptic seizures: Results from a prospective study. Epilepsy Behav. 2022;135:108890.
23. Duncan R, Oto M. Psychogenic nonepileptic seizures in patients with learning disability: comparison with patients with no learning disability. Epilepsy Behav. 2008;12(1):183-6.
24. Popkirov S, Grönheit W, Jungilligens J, Wehner T, Schlegel U, Wellmer J. Suggestive seizure induction for inpatients with suspected psychogenic nonepileptic seizures. Epilepsia. 2020;61(9):1931-8.
25. Benbadis SR. A spell in the epilepsy clinic and a history of "chronic pain" or "fibromyalgia" independently predict a diagnosis of psychogenic seizures. Epilepsy Behav. 2005;6(2):264-5.
26. Reuber M, Fernández G, Bauer J, Helmstaedter C, Elger CE. Diagnostic delay in psychogenic nonepileptic seizures. Neurology. 2002;58(3):493-5.
27. Avbersek A, Sisodiya S. Does the primary literature provide support for clinical signs used to distinguish psychogenic nonepileptic seizures from epileptic seizures? J Neurol Neurosurg Psychiatr. 2010;81(7):719-25.
28. Reuber M, Pukrop R, Mitchell AJ, Bauer J, Elger CE. Clinical significance of recurrent psychogenic nonepileptic seizure status. J Neurol. 2003;250(11):1355-62.
29. Syed TU, LaFrance WC Jr, Kahriman ES, Hasan SN, Rajasekaran V, Gulati D, et al. Can semiology predict psychogenic nonepileptic seizures? A prospective study. Ann Neurol. 2011;69(6):997-1004.
30. Whitehead K, Kane N, Wardrope A, Kandler R, Reuber M. Proposal for best practice in the use of video-EEG when psychogenic non-epileptic seizures are a possible diagnosis. Clin Neurophysiol Pract. 2017;2:130-9.
31. Popkirov S, Grönheit W, Wellmer J. A systematic review of suggestive seizure induction for the diagnosis of psychogenic nonepileptic seizures. Seizure. 2015;31:124-32.
32. Chen DK, T So Y, Fisher RS; Therapeutics and Technology Assessment Subcommittee of the American Academy of Neurology. Use of

prolactin in diagnosing epileptic seizures, Report of the therapeutics and technology assessment subcommittee of the American Academy of Neurology. Neurology. 2005;65(5):668-75.
33. Kerr WT, Janio EA, Chau AM, Braesch CT, Le JM, Hori JM, et al. Objective score from initial interview identifies patients with probable dissociative seizures. Epilepsy Behav. 2020;113:107525.
34. Baroni G, Martins WA, Rodrigues JC, Piccinini V, Marin C, de Lara Machado W, et al. A novel scale for suspicion of psychogenic nonepileptic seizures: development and accuracy. Seizure. 2021;89:65-72.
35. Lenio S, Kerr WT, Watson M, Baker S, Bush C, Rajic A, et al. Validation of a predictive calculator to distinguish between patients presenting with dissociative versus epileptic seizures. Epilepsy Behav. 2021;116:107767.
36. Dashtkoohi M, Ranji-Bourachaloo S, Pouremamali R, Dashtkoohi M, Zamani R, Moeinafshar A, et al. Clinical Functional Seizure Score (CFSS): a simple algorithm for clinicians to suspect functional seizures. Front Neurol. 2023;14:1295266.
37. LaFrance WC Jr, Reuber M, Goldstein LH. Management of psychogenic nonepileptic seizures. Epilepsia. 2013;54(Suppl 1):53-67.
38. Carton S, Thompson PJ, Duncan JS. Non-epileptic seizures: patients' understanding and reaction to the diagnosis and impact on outcome. Seizure. 2003;12(5):287-94.
39. Jalilianhasanpour R, Williams B, Gilman I, Burke MJ, Glass S, Fricchione GL, et al. Resilience linked to personality dimensions, alexithymia and affective symptoms in motor functional neurological disorders. J Psychosom Res. 2018;107:55-61.
40. Gasparini S, Beghi E, Ferlazzo E, Beghi M, Belcastro V, Biermann KP, et al. Management of psychogenic non-epileptic seizures: a multidisciplinary approach. Eur J Neurol. 2019;26(2):205-e15.
41. Carlson P, Perry KN. Psychological interventions for psychogenic non-epileptic seizures: A meta-analysis. Seizure. 2017;45:142-50.
42. LaFrance WC Jr, Miller IW, Ryan CE, Blum AS, Solomon DA, Kelley JE, et al. Cognitive behavioral therapy for psychogenic nonepileptic seizures. Epilepsy Behav. 2009;14:591-6.
43. Goldstein LH, Robinson EJ, Mellers JDC, Stone J, Carson A, Reuber M, et al.; CODES study group. Cognitive behavioural therapy for adults with dissociative seizures (CODES): a pragmatic, multicentre, randomised controlled trial. Lancet Psychiatry. 2020;7(6):491-505.
44. Myers L, Vaidya-Mathur U, Lancman M. Prolonged exposure therapy for the treatment of patients diagnosed with psychogenic non-epileptic seizures (PNES) and post-traumatic stress disorder (PTSD). Epilepsy Behav. 2017;66:86-92.
45. Howlett S, Reuber M. An augmented model of brief psychodynamic interpersonal therapy for patients with nonepileptic seizures. Psychotherapy (Chic). 2009;46(1):125-38.
46. LaFrance WC Jr, Alosco ML, Davis JD, Tremont G, Ryan CE, Keitner GI, et al. Impact of family functioning on quality of life in patients with psychogenic nonepileptic seizures versus epilepsy. Epilepsia. 2011;52(2):292-300.
47. Baslet G, Ridlon R, Raynor G, Gonsalvez I, Dworetzky BA. Sustained improvement with mindfulness-based therapy for psychogenic nonepileptic seizures. Epilepsy Behav. 2022;126:108478.
48. Zaroff CM, Myers L, Barr WB, Luciano D, Devinsky O. Group psychoeducation as treatment for psychological nonepileptic seizures. Epilepsy Behav. 2004;5(4):587-92.
49. Bajestan SN, Spiegel D, Barry JJ. Hypnosis for psychogenic nonepileptic seizures and psychogenic movement disorders. In: LaFrance, Jr WC, Schachter SC (Eds). Gates and Rowan's Nonepileptic Seizures, 4th edition. Cambridge: Cambridge University Press; 2018. pp. 90-8.
50. LaFrance WC, Baird GL, Barry JJ, Blum AS, Frank Webb A, Keitner GI, et al. Multicenter pilot treatment trial for psychogenic nonepileptic seizures: A randomized clinical trial. JAMA Psychiatry. 2014;71(9):997-1005.
51. Myers L, Sarudiansky M, Korman G, Baslet G. Using evidence-based psychotherapy to tailor treatment for patients with functional neurological disorders. Epilepsy Behav Rep. 2021;16:100478.
52. Tolchin B, Dworetzky BA, Martino S, Blumenfeld H, Hirsch LJ, Baslet G. Adherence with psychotherapy and treatment outcomes for psychogenic nonepileptic seizures. Neurology. 2019;92(7):e675-9.
53. Labiner DM, Bagic AI, Herman ST, Fountain NB, Walczak TS, Gumnit RJ; National Association of Epilepsy Centers. Essential services, personnel and facilities in specialized epilepsy centers-revised 2010 guidelines. Epilepsia. 2019;51(11):2322-33.
54. Hall-Patch L, Brown R, House A, Howlett S, Kemp S, Lawton G, et al. Acceptability and effectiveness of a strategy for the communication of the diagnosis

of psychogenic nonepileptic seizures. Epilepsia. 2010;51(1):70-8.
55. Bermeo-Ovalle A, Kanner A. The role of the neurologist after diagnosis. In: Dworetzky BA, Baslet G (Eds). Psychogenic Nonepileptic Seizures: Toward the Integration of Care. England: Oxford University Press; 2017. pp. 253-65.
56. Tolchin B, Dworetzky BA, Baslet G. Long-term adherence with psychiatric treatment among patients with psychogenic nonepileptic seizures. Epilepsia. 2018;59(1):e18-e22.
57. Whitehead K, Kandler R, Reuber M. Patients' and neurologists' perception of epilepsy and psychogenic nonepileptic seizures. Epilepsia. 2013;54(4):708-17.
58. Walther K, Volbers B, Erdmann L. Psychological long-term outcome in patients with psychogenic nonepileptic seizures. Epilepsia. 2019;60(4):669-78.
59. Durrant J, Rickards H, Cavanna AE. Prognosis and outcome predictors in psychogenic non-epileptic seizures. Epilepsy Res Treat. 2011;2011: 274736.

CHAPTER 11

Management of Genetic Epilepsies

Jyotsna AS, Bhargavi Sanji, KP Vinayan

ABSTRACT

With the advances in molecular genetics, understanding of genetic epilepsies and their underlying mechanisms have evolved tremendously, making a significant impact on the therapeutic decision-making. Subsequently, epilepsy management in children is slowly evolving from an epilepsy syndrome-based generic approach to an individually targeted approach, based on the underlying etiopathophysiologic mechanism. In this chapter, we present an overview of the current status of this ongoing paradigm shift in genetic epilepsies with a focus on those epilepsies that have an option of specific targeted treatments, which is of great relevance for neurological practice.

Keywords: Genetic epilepsies, Precision medicine, Epilepsy genes.

INTRODUCTION

Genetic epilepsies are estimated to constitute approximately one-third of all epilepsies.[1] The 2017 International League Against Epilepsy (ILAE) classification of epilepsies conceptually defines genetic epilepsy as an epilepsy that results directly from a known or presumed genetic mutation in which seizures are a core symptom of the disorder.[2] Pragmatically, a genetic etiology for epilepsy may be inferred in the situation of a strong family history (especially autosomal dominant inheritance) or by clinical research in populations with the same syndrome/ familial aggregation studies or when a genetic variant (single gene mutation/copy number/chromosomal aberration) is reproducibly associated with an epilepsy phenotype. Genetic epilepsies include epilepsies with monogenic (de novo or inherited pathogenic variants) or complex (polygenic with or without environmental factors) inheritance.[3]

The latest ILAE classification system proposed in 2022 describes epilepsy syndromes based on the age of onset, and genetic etiologies are enumerated under each epilepsy syndrome phenotype (e.g., infantile epileptic spasms syndrome and developmental/epileptic encephalopathy, etc.). Certain gene-specific epilepsy syndromes are also defined due to pathogenic variants in a single gene [e.g., *CDKL5* developmental and epileptic encephalopathy (CDKL5-DEE), *PCDH19* clustering epilepsy, glucose transporter 1 (GLUT1) deficiency syndrome—DEE and KCNQ2-DEE, etc.]. This chapter provides a brief overview of the current status of precision medicine in the epilepsies and suggests the adoption of a pragmatic approach.

Genetic generalized epilepsies are associated with a complex polygenic pattern as well as a significant environmental contribution. Moreover, structural focal epilepsies like focal cortical dysplasia (FCD) might also be associated with somatic mutations in the affected tissues. A detailed discussion on the management of both these syndromes with genetic underpinnings is beyond the scope of this chapter. Monogenic multiaxial neurological disorders (e.g., progressive myoclonus epilepsies) and multisystem diseases (e.g., lysosomal storage disorders) also may be viewed as a category of genetic epilepsy, though epilepsy may constitute only a part of the disease phenotype. Some of the diseases in this group are now amenable to targeted therapies. From the utilitarian perspective, this chapter will mention these disorders only if there is some role for precision medicine currently.

■ CLASSIFICATION OF GENETIC EPILEPSIES

Classification of genetic epilepsies may be approached in multiple ways. Pragmatically, a listing out of genes associated with various syndromes serves as a ready reckoner for a practicing neurologist. The major epilepsy syndromes and genes associated with them are enlisted in **Figure 1**. However,

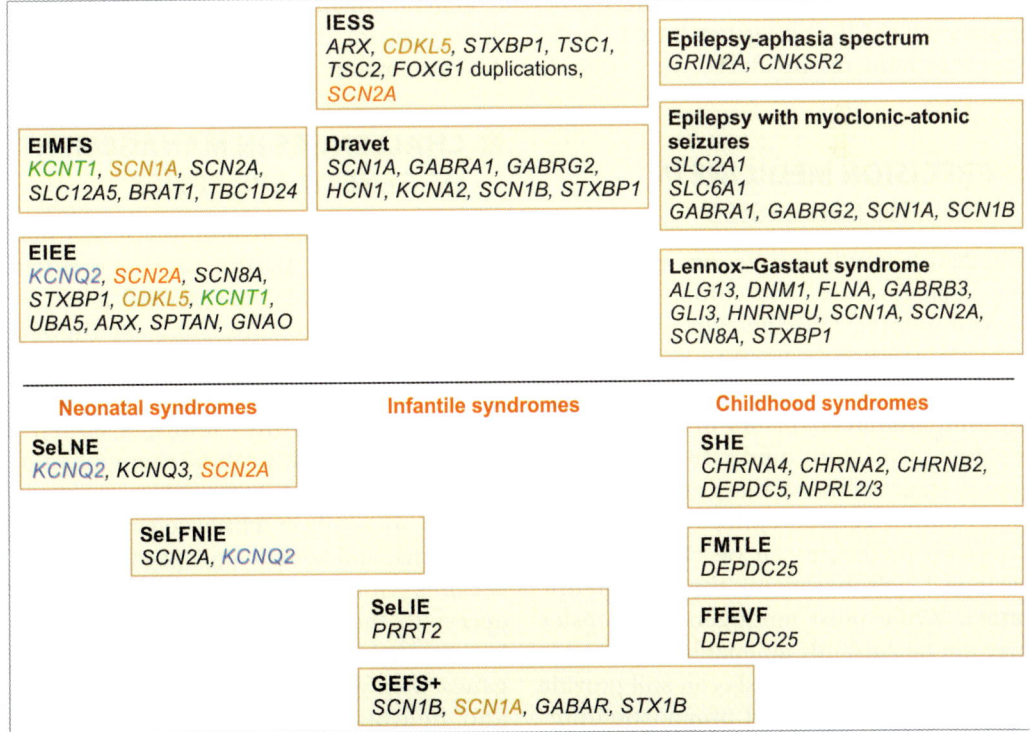

FIG. 1: Classification of genetic epilesies based on the electroclinical phenotype.
(EIEE: early infantile epileptic encephalopathy; EIMFS: epilepsy of infancy with migrating focal seizures; FFEVF: familial focal epilepsy with variable foci; FMTLE: familial mesial temporal lobe epilepsy; GEFS: genetic epilepsy with febrile seizures; IESS: infantile epileptic spasms syndrome; SHE: Sleep-related hypermotor epilepsy; SeLFNIE: self-limited familial neonatal-infantile epilepsy; SeLIE: self-limited infantile epilepsy; SeLNE: self-limited neonatal epilepsy)

TABLE 1: Classification of genetic epilepsies based on the etiopathology.

Pathomechanism	Examples
Ion channel or receptor defects	Sodium and potassium channel mutation-related epilepsies
Signaling pathway defects	m-TORopathies (tuberous sclerosis epilepsy)
Metabolic pathway defects	
Inborn errors of metabolism with epilepsy as a dominant/only phenotype	Pyridoxine-dependent epilepsy
Multiaxial neurological syndromes with epilepsy	Progressive myoclonus epilepsies and chromosomal disorders (ring chromosome 20-related epilepsy)
Multisystem disorders with epilepsy	Lysosomal storage diseases

(m-TOR: mammalian target of rapamycin)

from the perspective of understanding and management of genetic epilepsies, a classification by the pathomechanisms involved is more meaningful. **Table 1** gives an overview of the epilepsies based on the pathomechanisms involved, with suitable examples.

■ PRECISION MEDICINE IN GENETIC EPILEPSIES

"Precision medicine is an innovative approach that uses individual's genomic, environmental, and lifestyle information to guide decisions related to their medical management." With increasing knowledge on etiopathomechanisms of genetic epilepsies, precision medicine has taken center stage in the management of many well-defined genetic epilepsy syndromes. Precision medicine can be classified into various levels based on the therapeutic target. While most monogenic epilepsies may not be currently amenable to precision therapy, a proper diagnosis can still provide valuable phenotypic and prognostic information and can guide toward further evaluation and management (e.g., cardiac evaluation in *SCN1A*-associated Dravet syndrome and the use of sleep electroencephalography for detecting electrical status in sleep in *KCNB1*-related epileptic encephalopathy). **Figure 2** shows the tiers/levels in precision medicine, with examples of genetic epilepsies. In **Table 2**, the genetic epilepsies amenable to precision treatment are enumerated.

■ CHALLENGES IN MANAGEMENT OF GENETIC EPILEPSIES

Several challenges at multiple levels may be encountered in the management of genetic epilepsies. Phenotypic and genotypic heterogeneity is one such challenge. Phenotypic heterogeneity is where several types of mutations can occur in a single gene manifesting into multiple epilepsy phenotypes, and this can be exemplified by the *SCN1A* gene-related epilepsy spectrum which may result in febrile seizures, Dravet syndrome, and genetic epilepsy with febrile seizures (GEFS) plus phenotype.[4] Increased access to the next generation sequencing has resulted in the discovery of several such genes with a varied spectrum of epilepsy and neurological disorders.[5] Genotypic heterogeneity is when one epilepsy phenotype is associated with a number of different genes, which is best exemplified by the infantile epileptic spasms syndrome (IESS) that may be associated with multiple gene

CHAPTER 11: Management of Genetic Epilepsies

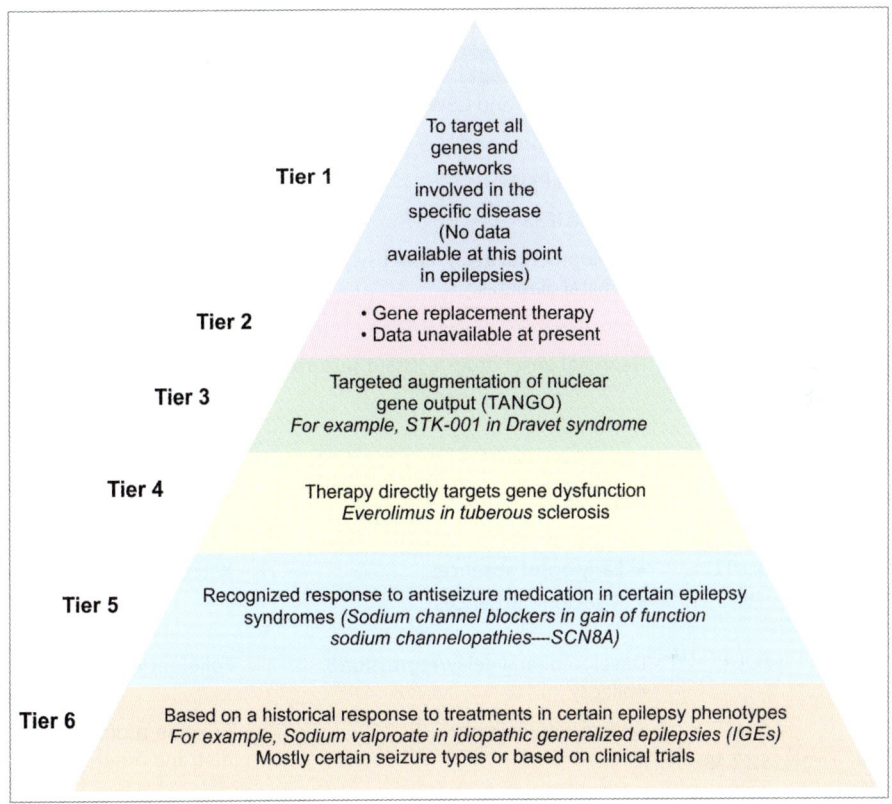

FIG. 2: Tiers/levels in precision medicine, with examples of genetic epilepsies.

TABLE 2: Genetic epilepsies amenable to precision treatment.

	Gene	Epilepsy syndrome	Treatment
Ion channels and receptors and others			
Sodium channel	SCN2A	• *Early onset:* BFNIE, DEE, and EIMFS—GoF • *Late onset:* Autism with seizures—LoF	• SCB: Phenytoin and CBZ • SCB may worsen
	SCN8A	• *Early onset:* Severe/moderate DEE and SeLFIE— GoF • *Late onset:* NDD with generalized epilepsy—LoF	• SCB: CBZ and OxCBZ • SCB: May worsen • *DOC:* Valproate, lamotrigine, and ethosuximide
	SCN1A	Dravet syndrome	• Valproate, clobazam, stiripentol, fenfluramine, and cannabidiols • Avoid SCB
Potassium channel	KCNQ2	BFNIE and DEE/EE	SCB and retigabine
	KCNT1	ADNFLE and EIMFS	Quinidine

Continued

Continued

	Gene	Epilepsy syndrome	Treatment
NMDA receptor	GRIN2A	SeLECTS, LKS, and CSWS	Memantine
	GRIN2B	West syndrome and LGS	Memantine
Others	PRRT2	SeLIE and PKD	SCB
	CDKL5	EIEE and IESS	Ganaxolone
	KATP	Developmental delay, epilepsy, and neonatal diabetes	Sulfonylurea
Inherited metabolic disorders			
Pyridoxine metabolism pathway	ALDH7A1	Neonatal onset drug-resistant seizures	• Pyridoxine ± folinic acid • Arginine, Lysine restricted diet
	PNPO		PLP ± Pyridoxine
Biotinidase deficiency	BTD	EIEE/DEE	Biotin
Glucose transporter deficiency	GLUT1	• Early onset absences • Myoclonic absences	Ketogenic diet
Cerebral folate deficiency	FOLR1	Developmental delay/regression ± epilepsy	Folinic acid
Creatine deficiency syndrome	GAMT SLC6A8 AGAT	Autism with epilepsy	Creatine, arginine-restricted diet, and ornithine
Serine biosynthesis disorders	3-PGDH PSAT PSP	Microcephaly and drug-resistant epilepsy	• Serine • Glycine
Folate metabolism	DHFR FR	Developmental delay and hypotonia	Folinic acid
Menkes disease	ATP7A	Progressive neurodegeneration	Copper histidine
CoQ10 (ubiquinone) deficiency syndromes	COQ2,4 PDSS1	Multisystem involvement	CoQ10
mTOR signaling pathways			
Tuberous sclerosis	TSC1/TSC2	Varied presentations	mTOR inhibitors: Everolimus
GATORopathies	DEPDC5 NPRL2 NPRL3	Lesional and nonlesional epilepsy	mTOR inhibitors: Everolimus

(ADNFLE: autosomal dominant nocturnal frontal lobe epilepsy; BFNIE: benign familial neonatal-infantile epilepsy; CBZ: carbamazepine; CSWS: continuous spikes and waves during sleep; DEE: developmental and epileptic encephalopathy; DOC: drug of choice; EIEE: early infantile epileptic encephalopathy; EIMFS: epilepsy of infancy with migrating focal seizures; EE: epileptic encephalopathy; GoF: gain-of-function; IESS: infantile epileptic spasms syndrome; LKS: Landau–Kleffner syndrome; LGS: Lennox–Gastaut syndrome; LoF: loss-of-function; NDD: neurodevelopmental disorders; NMDA: N-methyl-D-aspartate; PKD: paroxysmal kinesigenic dyskinesia; SCB: sodium channel blockers; SeLECTS: self-limited epilepsy with centrotemporal spikes; SeLFIE: self-limited infantile epilepsy) mutations like *KCNB1*, *KIF1A*, *SLC35A2*, *STXBP1*, *TBL1XR1*, and others.[6] **Figure 1** elucidates different epilepsy syndromes along with the associated genes. As a result, a specific mutation may not equate immediately to the diagnosis of a specific epilepsy syndrome. Furthermore, different pathogenic variants of the same gene can result in opposite functional effects, which has a bearing on the efficacy of therapy with certain classes of medication. A good example is *SCN2A*-related epilepsies where gain-of-function (GoF) mutations can be successfully treated with sodium channel blockers. On the contrary, sodium channel blockers may aggravate seizures related to loss-of-function (LoF) variants of the same *SCN2A* gene. Different mutations are known to cause different effects on the translated protein or downstream pathway, which may result in either a gain or loss of the protein's function.[7] Uncertainty in the pathogenicity of a mutation may lead to difficulties in decision-making and the answer to this problem may lie in the discovery of doable functional studies, which are still to evolve yet. A better understanding of the epileptic syndromes, the epilepsy genes, and the functional implications of their pathogenic variants are critical for the selection of antiseizure medication and also for development of novel therapies. In keeping with the explosion of information regarding the disease-causing genes, a periodic reevaluation of reported variants also is necessary at regular time intervals to deliver optimal patient care.

Cases 1 to 3 show illustrative examples of different types of genetic epilepsies and the vagaries in their presentation, natural history, and practical issues associated with decision-making.[8]

CASES

CASE 1

A 3-month-old baby with an uneventful perinatal period and normal development was brought with history of seizures from 10th day of life. The seizures as observed by the parents was of varied semiology. Predominantly, focal tonic and multifocal clonic type of seizures were described. EEG showed a normal background activity and sleep patterns. MRI was normal. The child had been initiated on levetiracetam and referred to a pediatric epilepsy center in the 3rd month of life in view of an abrupt increase in the seizure frequency to multiple daily brief seizures in a single week. Family history revealed similar seizures during infancy in the father and paternal uncle, which had abated by 2nd year of life. Oxcarbazepine was initiated, following which there was a complete cessation of seizures. Parents were anxious that the child may have recurrence of seizures and would watch the child through the night. NGS for epilepsy gene panel was sent, which showed a pathogenic variant in *SCN2A* gene. Parental segregation revealed the same variation in the father. Parents were counseled about the probability of self-limited nature of the child's epilepsy. It allayed the fear of withdrawal of antiseizure medication. Levetiracetam was withdrawn in 5th month of life. Oxcarbazepine was tapered off at 18 months of age. The child is presently developmentally normal and performing well at school.

(EEG: electroencephalogram; MRI: magnetic resonance imaging; NGS: Next-generation sequencing)

CASE 2

A 4-month-old baby girl, born to consanguineous parents, with uneventful perinatal period was brought with complaints of paroxysmal events from 2 weeks of life. Mother described shock-like jerks in clusters, especially on awakening. She had apparently lost social smile and her usual playfulness after the onset of the events. There was a family history of sibling death following severe developmental delay and epilepsy. On examination, child was noted to have poor visual fixation with a mild hypotonia. Patchy scalp alopecia noted. There were no other skin manifestations. The routine metabolic parameters were normal. Prolonged VEEG captured several habitual electroclinical events suggestive of epileptic spasms, and the interictal record was suggestive of modified hypsarrhythmia. MRI brain was normal. The child was initiated on ACTH therapy, and after a week, a 50% reduction in the spasm frequency was reported. Pyridoxine and valproate were initiated. Whole exome sequencing was done in view of it being a cryptogenic West syndrome, and it showed a likely pathogenic homozygous variant in *BTD* gene. She was initiated on biotin, and within a week, there was complete cessation of spasms. The child's developmental milestones also improved, but at the age of 3 years, she is yet to speak sentences, and walks with a mild unsteadiness of gait.

(ACTH: adrenocorticotropic hormone; MRI: magnetic resonance imaging; VEEG: video electroencephalogram)

CASE 3

A 3-year-old boy was referred to a pediatric epilepsy unit with history of absence seizures since 6 months, which persisted despite 3 antiseizure medications. He was born to nonconsanguineous parents with an uneventful perinatal period. The child was reported to have mild developmental delay when compared to the older sibling. There was no family history of seizures. Detailed probing into the seizure history revealed that the child had a few seizures in the past, which were suggestive of myoclonic and brief focal seizures, and these events had been noted specially in morning times. Parents also reported some unusual eye movements during infancy. Homemade videos of such events were noted to show rapid multidirectional eye movements accompanied by head movements in the same direction. The child's head size was less than third centile for age, while neurological examination was otherwise unremarkable. Video EEG captured multiple electroclinical events suggestive of atypical absence seizures. MRI brain was normal. Glucose transporter 1 (GLUT1) deficiency syndrome was suspected. CSF study revealed significant hypoglycorrhachia. Clinical exome sequencing showed a pathogenic mutation in *SLC2A1*, confirming the diagnosis of GLUT1 deficiency syndrome. Ketogenic diet was initiated which led to remarkable reduction in the seizure burden. However, the child's cognitive status continued to be subnormal for age, and during follow-up he was reported to be significantly below par in academic performance at school.

(CSF: cerebrospinal fluid; EEG: electroencephalogram; MRI: magnetic resonance imaging)

■ CONCLUSION

Marked expansion in the number of epilepsy-related genes has drastically impacted the outlook toward epilepsy therapeutics. This is well illustrated by precision medicine triumphs in some classically described genetic epilepsies (e.g., *ALDH7A1*-associated pyridoxine-dependent epilepsy and *SLC2A1*-associated GLUT1 deficiency syndrome). However, a successful treatment paradigm after genetic confirmation is not yet available for majority of genetic epilepsies. Better understanding of gene mutation–treatment response relationships will definitely help facilitate better selection of antiseizure medications.

REFERENCES

1. Hebbar M, Mefford HC. Recent advances in epilepsy genomics and genetic testing. F1000Res. 2020;9.
2. Scheffer IE, Berkovic S, Capovilla G, Connolly MB, French J, Guilhoto L, et al. ILAE Classification of the Epilepsies: Position Paper of the ILAE Commission for Classification and Terminology. Epilepsia. 2017;58(4):512-21.
3. Wirrell E, Tinuper P, Perucca E, Moshé SL. Introduction to the epilepsy syndrome papers. Epilepsia. 2022;63(6):1330-2.
4. Zuberi SM, Brunklaus A, Birch R, Reavey E, Duncan J, Forbes GH. Genotype-phenotype associations in SCN1A-related epilepsies. Neurology. 2011;76(7):594-600.
5. Symonds JD, Zuberi SM, Johnson MR. Advances in epilepsy gene discovery and implications for epilepsy diagnosis and treatment. Curr Opin Neurol. 2017;30(2):193-9.
6. Muir AM, Myers CT, Nguyen NT, Saykally J, Craiu D, De Jonghe P, et al. Genetic heterogeneity in infantile spasms. Epilepsy Res. 2019;156:106181.
7. Absalom NL, Liao VWY, Johannesen KMH, Gardella E, Jacobs J, Lesca G, et al. Gain-of-function and loss-of-function GABRB3 variants lead to distinct clinical phenotypes in patients with developmental and epileptic encephalopathies. Nat Commun. 2022;13:1822.
8. De Wachter M, Schoonjans AS, Weckhuysen S, Van Schil K, Löfgren A, Meuwissen M, et al. From diagnosis to treatment in genetic epilepsies: Implementation of precision medicine in real-world clinical practice. Eur J Paediatr Neurol. 2024;48:46-60.

CHAPTER 12

Management of Comorbidities of Epilepsy

Bindu Menon, Chandu Premkumar, Praveen Kumar Yadav

ABSTRACT

Comorbidity in persons with epilepsy is very high and diverse. Neurological, psychiatric, cognitive, cardiac, gastrointestinal (GI), somatic, and rheumatological conditions are identified more in persons with epilepsy than in the general population. In the present chapter, we discuss this issue in the context of common epilepsy comorbid conditions: Psychiatric comorbidity, cognitive impairment, attention-deficit hyperactivity disorder, migraine, GI, and endocrine disorders. Current findings, research limitations, and future directions of research efforts are discussed. The treatment of epilepsy requires comprehensive management of these associated conditions to ensure better patient outcomes and a higher quality of life. Optimal management involves multidisciplinary care and the ability to offer personalized treatment.

Keywords: Epilepsy, Comorbidities.

■ INTRODUCTION

Epilepsy is a chronic neurological disease affecting one in a hundred persons. Comorbidity in persons with epilepsy is very high and diverse. Neurological, psychiatric, cognitive, cardiac, gastrointestinal (GI), somatic and rheumatological conditions are identified more in persons with epilepsy than in the general population. Comorbidities can be a direct link as in patients with stroke. In yet other conditions like psychiatric comorbidities, the relationship could be more complex. Other comorbidities have no relationship as noted in cardiac conditions and could be coincidental. Identifying these comorbidities for comprehensive treatment and improving the quality of life is important.

The goal of epilepsy treatment is often seizure freedom. However, comprehensive care should also involve identifying and managing the comorbidities. Around half of the persons with epilepsy have at least one comorbidity. Larger population-based studies have noted this prevalence to be up to eight times more than the general population. As psychiatric comorbidities are more common, routine screening should be included in the long-term follow-up. The antiseizure medication (ASM) should also be tailored to address the comorbidities. With newer ASMs available, there are fewer pharmacokinetic and pharmacodynamic interactions with better tolerability. Here, we discuss the most common comorbidities of epilepsy in adults.

NEUROPSYCHIATRIC COMORBIDITY

Neurological and psychiatric comorbidities are common in people with epilepsy (PWE), affecting around 30–50% of patients.[1] According to population-based studies, the lifetime prevalence of psychiatric comorbidities is 35%, especially mood and anxiety disorders, while migraines are the most common neurological comorbidity, with a reported prevalence of 20–40%.[2,3]

Researchers agree that psychiatric disorders are more common in patients with epilepsy due to the availability of comprehensive epidemiological data on both adults and children with epilepsy.[4] The overall prevalence of active depression in epilepsy was 23.1%. There was an overall risk increase of 2.7 compared with the general population based on a meta-analysis of 14 population-based studies involving >1,000,000 adult participants.[5] A meta-analysis of 27 studies on anxiety disorders and epilepsy, involving >3,000 participants, found a combined prevalence of anxiety disorder at 20.2%. Generalized anxiety disorder was the most common, accounting for 10.2%.[6] In a meta-analysis of 57 studies involving over 40,000 participants, it was found the pooled prevalence of psychosis was 5.6% in unselected individuals, but it increased to 7% in temporal lobe epilepsy, and the pooled odds ratio for risk of psychosis among PWE compared with controls was 7.8.[7]

About 12% of PWE also experience psychogenic nonepileptic seizures (PNES) according to a meta-analysis. Additionally, 22% of those with PNES also have epilepsy.[8] Even though there is a strong emphasis on developmental disorders, data from pediatric epilepsy patients indicated no significant variances. According to a population-based study of 85 children and adolescents aged 5–15 years with active epilepsy, approximately 33% of the patients had attention deficit hyperactivity disorder (ADHD), 21% had autism spectrum disorder, 7% had depression, and 13% had anxiety.[9] The relationship between epilepsy and psychiatric disorders is complex, arising from a combination of psychosocial and biological factors. Epilepsy continues to be a highly stigmatized condition, leading to discrimination and marginalization.[10]

Patients with epilepsy often experience low self-esteem, social withdrawal, isolation, and distress due to challenges in social interaction, the unpredictability of seizures, and the potential for social embarrassment. Several biological factors contribute to the increased occurrence of psychiatric disorders in these individuals. Neuroimaging studies have found network abnormalities, particularly in the limbic structures, in patients with epilepsy and co-occurring depression.[10]

Various data from prospective observational studies have suggested that there is a bidirectional relationship between epilepsy and psychiatric disorders. Early death in individuals with epilepsy is associated with psychiatric comorbidities. Various factors, such as an increased risk of substance or alcohol abuse, a higher likelihood of injury, and elevated suicide rates can be possible causes.[10] There is a five-fold increased risk of sudden unexpected death in epilepsy (SUDEP) in female patients compared with those without such comorbidities as per the data from a nationwide population-based study.[11]

In primary and secondary care settings, screening tools are available for nearly all major psychiatric conditions in the general population. These tools are cost-effective as they are brief, standardized against the Diagnostic and Statistical Manual of Mental Disorders, Fifth Edition (DSM-5) criteria, and require fewer resources than a full clinical interview.[10]

The primary aim of any psychiatric intervention should always be to fully alleviate symptoms. However, there is limited current evidence on how to address psychiatric comorbidities in epilepsy. Nonetheless, there is no reason to believe that guidelines for treating psychiatric disorders on an international level may not apply to epilepsy. It is reasonable to follow psychiatric standards of care while taking into account the specific needs of individuals with epilepsy. This involves understanding the interactions between psychotropic drugs and ASMs, as well as the risk of seizures.[10]

There is a lack of literature about treatment options for individuals with epilepsy and psychiatric comorbidities. Studies have shown that selective serotonin reuptake inhibitors (SSRIs) and newer antidepressants can be used in PWE. Sertraline and citalopram are commonly used as first-line antidepressants for anxiety.[10] Different ASMs such as lamotrigine (LTG) and valproate (VPA) have various effects on mood. LTG has antidepressant effects, while VPA can lead to aggression. Certain antidepressants have been associated with an increased risk of seizures. ASMs such as phenytoin (PHT) and carbamazepine (CBZ) which induce enzymes, can lower the levels of antidepressants, while VPA and newer ASMs do not have the same effect. The connection between ASMs and suicide is not definitive. It is important to monitor side effects such as weight gain (with VPA and CBZ) and hyponatremia (with serotonin and norepinephrine reuptake inhibitors) in combination with CBZ, oxcarbazepine (OXC), and eslicarbazepine (ESL). Caution should be exercised with ASMs that have negative psychotropic effects such as benzodiazepines (BDZ), topiramate (TPM), and levetiracetam (LEV), while others such as LTG, lacosamide (LCM), pregabalin (PGB), and gabapentin are beneficial.[12]

■ COGNITIVE IMPAIRMENT

Patients with epilepsy often experience cognitive comorbidities that can impact their psychosocial functioning, education, career, emotional and social abilities, as well as overall well-being.[13]

Generally, patients with epilepsy frequently report difficulties with attention, executive functioning, and memory. Up to 70% of untreated patients found these issues before the onset of seizures or early in the diagnostic process.[14] These findings suggest shared mechanisms underlying cognitive and behavioral impairments, as well as seizures in individuals with epilepsy, known as essential comorbidities. Seizure activity in epilepsy can temporarily lead to cognitive impairment. Cognitive impairment may be due to interictal spikes, the adverse effects of ASMs, and can be made worse by mood and behavioral issues. In the DSM-5, having an intellectual disability is generally defined as having a full-scale intelligence quotient (IQ) of ≤65–75, indicating cognitive functioning that is significantly below the population average of 100.[10]

Psychiatric and behavioral issues are 2.5 times more common in children with epilepsy than in their healthy peers. This can be challenging in persons with moderate-to-severe intellectual disabilities due to behavioral issues such as aggression or self-injurious behaviors.[10]

Notable developmental delays, intellectual disabilities, and severe, drug-resistant epilepsy occur in many childhood epilepsy syndromes.[15] These conditions are often referred to as developmental epileptic encephalopathies and include syndromes such as Lennox–Gastaut syndrome and Landau–Kleffner syndrome.

Dementia is an increasingly important cognitive comorbidity of epilepsy. Dementia and epilepsy have a bidirectional relationship, with an increased risk of seizures among those with dementia and an increased risk of dementia for those with epilepsy. To emphasize the importance of understanding cognitive comorbidities in epilepsy, individuals with epilepsy and intellectual disabilities are at a greater risk of developing dementia compared to those with epilepsy but without intellectual disabilities.[16]

For the diagnosis of cognitive comorbidity and the identification of patients who require more detailed neuropsychological assessment, cognitive screening measures such as the montreal cognitive assessment (MoCA) or mini-mental state examination (MMSE) can be useful.

A formal neuropsychological assessment is a collaborative and holistic process that takes into account biological, neurodevelopmental, psychological, and broader social factors. It is essential for accurately diagnosing cognitive deficits.[10]

Only a few studies have looked at how well medications or neuromodulatory interventions improve cognition, even though a lot of research on cognitive issues in epilepsy is available. Noninvasive neuromodulation for epilepsy is attractive because it could potentially reduce seizure frequency and interictal epileptiform discharge frequency, but there is still limited data on its effects on cognition.[17]

Compared to other types of dementia, epilepsy in Alzheimer's disease (AD) may respond better to ASMs as per a few studies. A thorough discussion with patients and their families and careful weighing of the risks and benefits of undergoing surgery is required, when surgical treatment is considered for epilepsy.[10]

An increasing body of research indicates that modified therapeutic approaches, such as cognitive behavioral therapy (CBT), can be effective in treating anxiety and depression in patients with cognitive impairments.[18] The relationship between AD and epilepsy is not well understood. Preclinical models of AD are important for studying the connections between AD and epilepsy and for developing new ASMs. Limited research exists on ASMs in preclinical models of late-onset epilepsy, and more high-quality randomized controlled trials (RCTs) are needed to determine the therapeutic efficacy of ASMs in AD. Future research should focus on AD patients with subclinical epileptiform activity and utilize tools like video electroencephalogram (EEG) to identify those who might benefit from ASMs.[19]

■ SLEEP DISORDERS

In persons with epilepsy, sleep disorders are around twice as common compared to healthy controls, and about one-third of PWE report a disturbance in their sleep.[20] Insomnia is common in PWE, with an estimated prevalence of up to 50%.[20] About 10–35% of individuals with epilepsy also experience comorbid obstructive sleep apnea (OSA), and a significantly higher incidence of OSA in those with refractory seizures.[21] With a possible prevalence of up to 89%, OSA seems to be more prevalent in older patients and late-onset epilepsy.[21] In elderly patients, OSA is likely to promote seizure occurrence.[21]

An increased prevalence of OSA in epilepsy is linked to several factors, such as a higher incidence of metabolic syndrome. This is influenced by reduced physical activity and weight-gaining ASMs like VPA.[22] In 28–57% of patients, vagal nerve stimulation (VNS) can also trigger or worsen OSA possibly by inducing adduction of the left vocal cord.[22]

In PWE, excessive daytime sleepiness affects 11–34% of individuals, and 13% experience restless leg syndrome (RLS).[23]

All of these disorders are approximately twice as common in PWE, than in the control group, with odds ratios ranging from 1.7 for insomnia to 4.7 for RLS in epilepsy patients compared to controls.[24,25]

The PWE often experience changes in their sleep patterns, not only because of seizures during the night. Those with juvenile myoclonic epilepsy (JME) tend to have lower sleep efficiency, less non-rapid eye movement (REM) sleep, reduced time in REM sleep, and increased wakefulness compared to those without epilepsy.[21]

A lack of sleep at night could raise the likelihood of experiencing seizures during the day and night. Mental health issues and difficulties with thinking for PWE result from a cycle of seizures and sleep problems which ultimately reduce their overall quality of life.[21]

The study findings imply that gamma-aminobutyric acid (GABA) enhancers (specifically tiagabine), calcium-channel blockers (like CBZ), synaptic vesicle protein 2A (SV2A) ligands (like LEV), and broad-spectrum ASMs did not have an impact on slow wave sleep (SWS), REM sleep, or sleep efficiency.[26] The impact of ASMs on sleep remains poorly investigated in PWE till date.[27]

When sleep disorders are suspected, diagnostic tests such as actigraphy, home sleep testing, and polysomnography (PSG) are generally recommended by clinical practice guidelines. These recommendations apply to both people with stable epilepsy and those without epilepsy. Individuals with nonstable forms of epilepsy should undergo inpatient or ambulatory video-PSG with extended EEG coverage. This is considered appropriate for diagnosing sleep-disordered breathing (SDB) and other comorbid sleep disorders, as well as for identifying unreported nocturnal epileptic seizures that may contribute to sleep disruption.[21] First-generation ASM, including barbiturates, BDZ, PHT, and phenobarbital (PB), have been found to decrease the duration of REM and SWS. These medications have the potential to impact the quality and duration of sleep due to their effects on REM and SWS patterns. BDZ, LTG, LEV, gabapentin, and PGB are known to increase sleep efficiency. Cannabidiol (CBD) can control drop attacks, and cannabis may have therapeutic benefits for sleep but can also negatively impact sleep after withdrawal. Continuous positive airway pressure (CPAP) therapy is an effective method for treating OSA and improving oxygen saturation levels during sleep.[28]

■ MIGRAINE

Migraine and epilepsy are neurological disorders that share similar paroxysmal clinical manifestations, yet migraine is a more prevalent episodic neurological disorder. The prevalence of migraine in populations of individuals with epilepsy is estimated at 8–24%.[29-31]

The co-occurrence of epilepsy in people with migraine ranges from 1 to 17% with a median prevalence of 5.9%, significantly higher than the general population being 0.5–1%. Epilepsy being a complex disorder than migraine is often accompanied by a range of co-occurring comorbidities. Epilepsy not only carries its challenges but also poses a risk for developing comorbid conditions such as depression, anxiety, dementia, migraine, heart disease, and peptic ulcer disease, with a prevalence up to eight times higher than the general population.

Migraine is thought to be triggered by a phenomenon known as cortical spreading depression (CSD), which involves a wave of cellular hyperexcitability and depolarization in the brain. In contrast, epilepsy results from abnormal hypersynchronous electrical activity within specific brain circuits.[32-34] Glutamate, the primary excitatory neurotransmitter in the brain plays a central role in the pathophysiology of both migraine and epilepsy. In epilepsy, α-amino-3-hydroxy-5-methyl-4-isoxazolepropionic acid (AMPA) receptor-mediated neuronal excitability leads to seizures. In migraine on the other hand, it is thought to induce migraine attacks by activating N-methyl-D-aspartate (NMDA) receptors, which causes hyperexcitability in the trigeminovascular system and the dura mater.[35]

There is a strong genetical association between epilepsy and familial hemiplegic migraine (FHM), of these *CACNA1*, *ATP1A2*, *SCN1A*, and *PRRT2* are the four genes involved in genetic mutation. A common genetic thread links epilepsy, FHM, and a specific mutation in the *CACNA1* gene. This mutation can be found in patients with either epilepsy or FHM alone, as well as in those with both conditions existing concurrently as comorbidities.[36]

The ASM exerts antimigraine activity by attenuating neurogenic inflammation in the trigeminal vascular system by preventing the release of calcitonin gene-related peptide (CGRP), and other vasoactive peptides and blocking CSD and preventing central sensitization, which are responsible for triggers of migraine. ASMs that are approved for migraine prophylaxis and epilepsy are sodium VPA/divalproex sodium maximum of 500–1,000 mg/day and TPM maximum of 100 mg/day with low titration.[37-39]

While not conventionally used as migraine prophylaxis ASMs such as LTG, zonisamide, gabapentin, PGB, CBZ, and LEV, are effective in the management of migraine with aura, particularly when conventional migraine prophylactics fail.

Women with childbearing potential are recommended to avoid VPA and CBZ which is highly potential to cause major congenital malformation and neurodevelopmental disorders.

■ GASTROINTESTINAL SYSTEM

The GI system communicates to the Brain via vagus nerve fibers and the gut-brain axis.[40] This network is maintained by gut microbiota and neurotransmitter substances such as serotonin, immune-mediated release of cytokines, interleukin-1β, and tumor necrosis factor alpha (TNF-α) via afferent neuronal messages from the enteric nervous system (ENS).[40,41] Approximately 0.7–9.1% of patients with celiac disease and irritable bowel syndrome (IBS) are known to cause epilepsy.[42,43] Immune-mediated mechanism, vitamin B12 and thiamine deficiency are implicated in the pathogenesis of epileptic seizures in immune-mediated GI disorders.[44] ASMs have no major role in GI-induced epilepsy mainly for celiac and IBS. Many drugs have been avoided mainly due to their side effect profile such as abdominal cramps, nausea, vomiting, weight loss, and hepatotoxicity in drugs such as valproic acid, ethosuximide, TPM, and felbamate.[44-47] The mainstay of treatment in these conditions is immunomodulatory drugs. The ketogenic and gluten-free diet has been beneficial for curing celiac disease.[48]

■ FIBROMYALGIA

Fibromyalgia is a chronic pain disorder, causing pain and tenderness throughout the body as well as fatigue and insomnia, affecting 2% of the population. Among patients with fibromyalgia, 11% had epileptic seizures, 74% had psychogenic nonepileptic events, and 15% had psychological nonepileptic events.[49] PNES is most seen in association with fibromyalgia and self-limiting seizures. The mechanism postulated is the discomfort produced in chronic pain which causes psychological distress and PNES.[50] ASMs that are approved for fibromyalgia and chronic low backache are gabapentin and PGB with less side effect profile.[51] Other ASMs including CBZ, clobazam, PHT, and VPA have no or insufficient evidence of effect.[50-51]

■ ENDOCRINE DISORDERS

Thyroid hormones play an essential role in the maintenance of central nervous system development, myelination, and physiological functions. Thyroid hormones are necessary to maintain mitochondrial brain function, modulate the development and function of GABAergic interneurons, and regulate the brain's antioxidant properties.[52]

Epilepsy is one of the most common neurological disorders affecting people of all ages, and the pathogenesis behind thyroid hormone functions and epilepsy share similar mechanisms.[53] Epilepsy is caused by the failure in regulation of excitatory neurotransmitter (glutamate) and inhibitory (GABA) amino acids in the brain, along with oxidative stress and mitochondrial dysfunction.[54]

Polytherapy specifically CBZ, OXC, PHT, VPA, and PB treatment has been shown to reduce thyroid hormones and lead to hypothyroidism and its related disease-related complications.[55]

REPRODUCTIVE ENDOCRINE DISORDER INCLUDING POLYCYSTIC OVARY SYNDROME

Epilepsy is associated with reproductive endocrine disorders like polycystic ovary syndrome (PCOS), isolated components of this syndrome such as polycystic ovaries, hypothalamic amenorrhea, and hyperprolactinemia. The mechanism behind endocrine disorders and epilepsy postulated are the direct effect of ASMs, enzyme-inducing agents such as CBZ and PHT on endocrine control centers in the brain mainly the hypothalamic-pituitary-adrenal axis.[56] Patients on VPA should be cautious of PCOS and weight gain, there can be menstrual disturbance, fertility issues, hirsutism, and galactorrhea in patients on VPA.[56]

If women with PCOS and reproductive endocrine disorders are found, antiepileptic drug treatment should be reviewed to ensure whether the drug is accurate for a particular seizure type.[56]

CARDIOVASCULAR SYSTEM

Cardiovascular diseases cause a major risk of mortality in patients with epilepsy.[57] Cardiovascular risk factors such as obesity, diabetes, hypertension, and hyperlipidemia have a direct association with epilepsy and are considered the major cause of death in PWE.[58,59]

The incidence ratio of heart disease to stroke in epilepsy is (3.54-4.9) for heart disease and (4.19-5.84.) for stroke respectively.[60] Among cardiovascular disorders incidence of myocardial infarction (MI) is around 2.34-10.1 and mortality due to MI is higher as compared to the general population.[61] Older ASMs such as PHT, PB, and CBZ are hepatic enzyme inducers associated with vascular risks. Fosphenytoin is safer when compared to PHT with a lower incidence of hypotension and lesser tissue side effects. VPA and LTG are generally well tolerated. The newer ASM, LCM has cardiac effects with rapid intravenous dosing and is associated with first-degree atrioventricular (AV) block in less than one-fourth of the patients.[62]

HYPERTENSION AND DIABETES

Hypertension and diabetes are some of the vascular risk factors for late-onset epilepsy. Patients with preexisting cardiovascular disorders, arrhythmias, and heart failures are at high risk of SUDEP. Heart rate variability during seizures is the reason underlying SUDEP; reduced heart rate variability is associated with risk of cardiac mortality from arrhythmias and sudden cardiac death.[63,64]

During prolonged seizures especially during generalized tonic-clonic seizures (GTCS), the vagus nerve acts to reduce heart rate via sinoatrial (SA) and AV node by protecting the heart from hypoxia, ischemia, and stress.

Mechanisms underlying the association between epilepsy and cardiovascular disease include the adverse effects of enzyme-inducing ASMs on cholesterol, lipid metabolism, and obesity, lifestyle habits such as increased smoking and decreased physical activity in persons with epilepsy. Chronic epilepsy itself has adverse effects on the heart.

CONCLUSION

The treatment of epilepsy requires comprehensive management of the associated conditions to ensure better patient outcomes and a higher quality of life. Optimal management involves multidisciplinary care and the ability to offer personalized treatment. Both pharmacological and nonpharmacological treatments need to be considered. Patient education is essential to ensure treatment adherence.

REFERENCES

1. Gaitatzis A, Carroll K, Majeed A, W Sander J. The epidemiology of the comorbidity of epilepsy in the general population. Epilepsia. 2004;45(12):1613-22.
2. Tellez-Zenteno JF, Patten SB, Jetté N, Williams J, Wiebe S. Psychiatric comorbidity in epilepsy: a population-based analysis. Epilepsia. 2007; 48(12):2336-44.
3. Hesdorffer DC, Lúdvígsson P, Hauser WA, Olafsson E, Kjartansson O. Co-occurrence of major depression or suicide attempt with migraine with aura and risk for unprovoked seizure. Epilepsy Res. 2007;75(2-3):220-3.
4. Salpekar JA, Mula M. Common psychiatric comorbidities in epilepsy: How big of a problem is it? Epilepsy Behav. 2019;98(Pt B):293-7.
5. Fiest KM, Dykeman J, Patten SB, Wiebe S, Kaplan GG, Maxwell CJ, et al. Depression in epilepsy: a systematic review and meta-analysis. Neurology. 2013;80(6):590-9.
6. Scott AJ, Sharpe L, Hunt C, Gandy M. Anxiety and depressive disorders in people with epilepsy: A meta-analysis. Epilepsia. 2017;58(6):973-82.
7. Clancy MJ, Clarke MC, Connor DJ, Cannon M, Cotter DR. The prevalence of psychosis in epilepsy; a systematic review and meta-analysis. BMC Psychiatry. 2014;75:14.
8. Kutlubaev MA, Xu Y, Hackett ML, Stone J. Dual diagnosis of epilepsy and psychogenic nonepileptic seizures: Systematic review and meta-analysis of frequency, correlates, and outcomes. Epilepsy Behav. 2018;89:70-8.
9. Reilly C, Atkinson P, Das KB, Chin RF, Aylett SE, Burch V, et al. Neurobehavioral comorbidities in children with active epilepsy: a population-based study. Pediatrics. 2014;133(6):e1586-93.
10. Mula M, Coleman H, Wilson SJ. Neuropsychiatric and cognitive comorbidities in epilepsy. Continuum (Minneap Minn). 2022;28(2):457-82.
11. Sveinsson O, Andersson T, Carlsson S, Tomson T. The incidence of SUDEP: A nationwide population-based cohort study. Neurology. 2017;89(2):170-7.
12. Trimble MR, Mula M. Antiepileptic drug interactions in patients requiring psychiatric drug treatment. In: Majkowski J, Bourgeois BFD, Patsalos PN, Mattson RH, Lam E, Routledge PA, et al. (Eds). Antiepileptic Drugs. Cambridge: Cambridge University Press; 2005. pp. 350-68.
13. Quintas R, Raggi A, Giovannetti AM, Pagani M, Sabariego C, Cieza A, et al. Psychosocial difficulties in people with epilepsy: a systematic review of literature from 2005 until 2010. Epilepsy Behav. 2012;25(1):60-7.
14. Witt JA, Helmstaedter C. Cognition in epilepsy: current clinical issues of interest. Curr Opin Neurol. 2017;30(2):174-9.
15. Kaga M, Inagaki M, Ohta R. Epidemiological study of Landau-Kleffner syndrome (LKS) in Japan. Brain Dev. 2014;36(4):284-6.
16. Robertson J, Hatton C, Emerson E, Baines S. Prevalence of epilepsy among people with intellectual disabilities: A systematic review. Seizure. 2015;29:46-62.
17. Jacobs CS, Willment KC, Sarkis RA. Non-invasive Cognitive Enhancement in Epilepsy. Front Neurol. 2019;10:167.
18. Ponsford J, Lee NK, Wong D, McKay A, Haines K, Downing M, et al. Factors associated with

response to adapted cognitive behavioral therapy for anxiety and depression following traumatic brain injury. J Head Trauma Rehabil. 2020;35(2):117-26.
19. del Pozo A, Lehmann L, Knox KM, Barker-Haliski M. Can old animals reveal new targets? The aging and degenerating brain as a new precision medicine opportunity for epilepsy. Front Neurol. 2022;13:833624.
20. van Golde EG, Gutter T, de Weerd AW. Sleep disturbances in people with epilepsy; prevalence, impact and treatment. Sleep Med Rev. 2011;15(6):357-68.
21. Nobili L, Beniczky S, Eriksson SH, Romigi A, Ryvlin P, Toledo M, et al. Expert Opinion: Managing sleep disturbances in people with epilepsy. Epilepsy Behav. 2021;124:108341.
22. Söylemez E, Öztürk O, Baslo SA, Balçık ZE, Ataklı D. Metabolic syndrome and obstructive sleep apnea syndrome among patients with epilepsy on monotherapy. Epilepsy Behav. 2020;111:107296.
23. Lowe CJ, Safati A, Hall PA. The neurocognitive consequences of sleep restriction: A meta-analytic review. Neurosci Biobehav Rev. 2017;80:586-604.
24. Gammino M, Zummo L, Bue AL, Urso L, Terruso V, Marrone O, et al. Excessive daytime sleepiness and sleep disorders in a population of patients with epilepsy: a case-control study. J Epilepsy Res. 2016;6(2):79-86.
25. Lin Z, Si Q, Xiaoyi Z. Obstructive sleep apnoea in patients with epilepsy: a meta-analysis. Sleep Breath. 2017;21(2):263-70.
26. Yeh WC, Lu SR, Wu MN, Lee KW, Chien CF, Fong YO, et al. The impact of antiseizure medications on polysomnographic parameters: a systematic review and meta-analysis. Sleep Med. 2021;81:319-26.
27. Romigi A, Cappellano S, Caccamo M, Testa F, Centonze D. The impact of antiseizure medications on polysomnographic parameters: a systematic review and meta-analysis. Sleep Med. 2021;88:290.
28. Choi S, Huang BC, Gamaldo CE. Therapeutic uses of cannabis on sleep disorders and related conditions. J Clin Neurophysiol. 2020;37(1):39-49.
29. Toldo I, Perissinotto E, Menegazzo F, Boniver C, Sartori S, Salviati L, et al. Comorbidity between headache and epilepsy in a pediatric headache center. J Headache Pain. 2010;11:235-40.
30. Ottman R, Lipton RB. Comorbidity of migraine and epilepsy. Neurology. 1994;44:2105-10.
31. Haut SR, Bigal ME, Lipton RB. Chronic disorders with episodic manifestations: focus on epilepsy and migraine. Lancet Neurol. 2006;5(2):148-57.
32. Trevelyan AJ, Sussillo D, Yuste R. Feedforward inhibition contributes to the control of epileptiform propagation speed. J Neurosci. 2007;27(13):3383-7.
33. Yamaguchi S, Donevan SD, Rogawski MA. Anticonvulsant activity of AMPA/kainate antagonists: comparison of GYKI 52466 and NBOX in maximal electroshock and chemoconvulsant seizure models. Epilepsy Res. 1993;15(3):179-84.
34. Pietrobon D, Moskowitz MA. Chaos and commotion in the wake of cortical spreading depression and spreading depolarizations. Nat Rev Neurosci. 2014;15(6):379-93.
35. Jasper HH, Ward A, Pope A. In: Noebels JL, Avoli M, Rogawski MA, Olsen RW, Delgado-Escueta AV (Eds). Jasper's Basic Mechanisms of Epilepsies, 4th Edition. Bethesda (MD): National Center for Biotechnology Information (US); 2012.
36. Rogawski MA. Migraine and epilepsy-shared mechanisms within the family of episodic disorders. In: Noebels JL, Avoli M, Rogawski MA, Olsen RW, Delgado-Escueta AV, (Eds). Jasper's Basic Mechanisms of the Epilepsies. Bethesda, MD: National Center for Biotechnology Information (US); 2012.
37. Calabresi P, Galletti F, Rossi C, Sarchielli P, Cupini LM. Antiepileptic drugs in migraine: From clinical aspects to cellular mechanisms. Trends Pharmacol Sci. 2007;28(4):188-95.
38. Frank F, Ulmer H, Sidoroff V, Broessner G. CGRP-antibodies, topiramate and botulinum toxin type A in episodic and chronic migraine: A systematic review and meta-analysis. Cephalalgia. 2021;41(11-12):1222-39.
39. Zobdeh F, Kraiem A, Attwood MM, Chubarev VN, Tarasov VV, Schiöth HB, et al. Pharmacological treatment of migraine: Drug classes, mechanisms of action, clinical trials and new treatments. Br J Pharmacol. 2021;178(23):4588-607.
40. Mittal R, Debs LH, Patel AP, Nguyen D, Patel K, Hamed G, et al. Neurotransmitters: The critical modulators regulating gut-brain axis: HHS public access. J Cell Physiol. 2017;232(9):2359-72.
41. Pfeiffer RF. Gastroenterology and neurology. Continuum: Lifelong Learning in Neurology. 2017;23(3):744-61.
42. Işikay S, Kocamaz H. Prevalence of celiac disease in children with idiopathic epilepsy in Southeast Turkey. Pediatr Neurol. 2014;50(5):479-81.
43. Djuric Z, Nagorni A, Jocic-Jakubi B, Dimic M, Novak M, Milicevic R, et al. Celiac disease prevalence in epileptic children from Serbia. Turk J Pediatr. 2012;54(3):247.

44. Casella G, Tontini GE, Bassotti G, Pastorelli L, Villanacci V, Spina L, et al. Neurological disorders and inflammatory bowel diseases. World J Gastroenterol. 2014;20(27):8764-82.
45. Powell-Jackson PR, Tredger JM, Williams R. Hepatotoxicity to sodium valproate: A review. Gut. 1984;25(6):673-81.
46. Dreifuss FE, Langer DH. Side effects of valproate. Am J Med. 1988;84(1A):34-41
47. O'Neil MG, Perdun CS, Wilson MB, McGown ST, Patel S. Felbamate-associated fatal acute hepatic necrosis. Neurology. 1996;46(5):1457-9.
48. Pratesi R, Modelli IC, Martins RC, Almeida PL, Gandolfi L. Celiac disease and epilepsy: Favorable outcome in a child with difficult to control seizures. Acta Neurologica Scandinavica. 2003;108(4):290-3.
49. Tatum WO, Langston ME, Acton EK. Fibromyalgia and seizures. Epileptic Disord. 2016;18(2):148-54.
50. Benbadis SR. A spell in the epilepsy clinic and a history of "chronic pain" or "fibromyalgia" independently predict a diagnosis of psychogenic seizures. Epilepsy Behav. 2005;6:264-5.
51. Wiffen PJ, Derry S, Moore RA, Aldington D, Cole P, Rice AS, et al. Antiepileptic drugs for neuropathic pain and fibromyalgia–an overview of cocrane reviews. Cochrane Database Syst Rev. 2013;2013(11):CD010567.
52. Tamijani SMS, Karimi B, Amini E, Golpich M, Dargahi L, Ali RA, et al. Thyroid hormones: possible roles in epilepsy pathology. Seizure. 2015;31:155-64.
53. Veliskova J, Desantis KA. Sex and hormonal influences on seizures and epilepsy. Horm Behav. 2013;63(2):267-77.
54. Chang SJ, Yu BC. Mitochondrial matters of the brain: mitochondrial dysfunction and Oxidative status in epilepsy. J Bioenerg Biomembr. 2010;42(6):457-9.
55. Lai EC, Yang YH, Lin SJ, Hsieh CY. Use of anti-epileptic drug and risk of hypothyroidism. Pharmacoepidemiol Drug Saf. 2013;22(10):1071-9.
56. Isojärvi JI. Reproductive dysfunction in women with epilepsy. Neurology. 2003;61(6 Suppl 2):S27-34.
57. Gaertner ML, Mintzer S, DeGiorgio CM. Increased cardiovascular risk in epilepsy. Front Neurol. 2024;15:1339276.
58. DeGiorgio CM, Curtis A, Carapetian A, Hovsepian D, Krishnadasan A, Markovic D. Why are epilepsy mortality rates rising in the United States? A population-based multiple cause-of-death study. BMJ Open. 2020;10(8):e035767.
59. DeGiorgio CM, Curtis AT, Hertling D, Kerr WT, Markovic D. Changes in epilepsy causes of death: a US population study. Acta Neurol Scand. 2021;144(5):478-85.
60. Chen Z, Liew D, Kwan P. Excess mortality and hospitalized morbidity in newly treated epilepsy patients. Neurology. 2016;87:718-25.
61. Janszky I, Hallqvist J, Tomson T, Ahlbom A, Mukamal KJ, Ahnve S. Increased risk and worse prognosis of myocardial infarction in patients with prior hospitalization for epilepsy–the Stockholm Heart Epidemiology Program. Brain. 2009;132:2798-804.
62. Lu Y-T, Lin C-H, Ho C-J, Hsu C-W, Tsai M-H. Evaluation of Cardiovascular Concerns of Intravenous Lacosamide Therapy in Epilepsy Patients. Front Neurol. 2022;13:891368.
63. Galinier M, Pathak A, Fourcade J, Androdias C, Curnier D, Varnous S, et al. Depressed low frequency power of heart rate variability as an independent predictor of sudden death in chronic heart failure. Eur Heart J. 2000;21:475-82.
64. Shah SA, Kambur T, Chan C, Herrington DM, Liu K, Shah SJ. Relation of short-term heart rate variability to incident heart failure (from the Multi-Ethnic Study of Atherosclerosis). Am J Cardiol. 2013;112:533-40.

Index

Page numbers followed by *b* refer to box, *f* refer to figure, *fc* refer to flowchart, and *t* refer to table.

A

Alcohol 94
Alexithymia 111*f*
Alpha-amino-3-hydroxy-5-methyl-4-isoxazolepropionic acid 33, 134
  receptor 95
Alpha-aminoadipic semialdehyde 104
Altered movement, paroxysmal episodes of 109
Alzheimer's disease 10, 133
American Academy of Neurology 3, , 82
Anesthesia 100
Anesthetic
  agents 96
  cycles
    cycling of 100
    duration of 100
  medications 96, 97*t*
    choice of 100
  speed of weaning of 100
Antiepileptic drugs 68, 82
  new 45
Antiseizure medications 3, 5, 6, 11, 17, 19, 30, 31, 35, 36*t*, 38*b*, 40, 48, 49*t*, 51, 55-59, 62, 66, 89, 94, 109, 112, 117, 130, 200
  balancing 20*fc*
  choice 34
  clinical trials of 14
  combination 37
  discontinuation of 117
  management 41
  number of 52
  role of 31
  salient features of 59*b*
  serum level of 52
  withdrawal 49, 49*b*, 50-52, 52*t*, 54, 55
  following surgery, timing of 53
  speed of 53
  timing of 53
Anxiety 24, 111, 134
  disorder
    generalized 25
    social 25
Aphasia 65
  postictal 66
Arginine 126
Atkin's diet, modified 45, 75
Atrioventricular block 136
Attacks, nonepileptic 110
Attention-deficit hyperactivity disorder 23, 131
Auditory hallucinations 65
Aura 64
Autism spectrum disorder 22
Autoimmune panel 94
Autosomal dominant nocturnal frontal lobe epilepsy 126

B

Barbiturates 97
Benign familial neonatal-infantile epilepsy 126
Benzodiazepine 32, 95, 132
Biotin 126
Biotinidase deficiency 126
Bipolar disorder 25
Birth rates 24
Bone
  health 24
  marrow suppression 36
Brain tumors, low-grade 73
Breathing
  sleep disordered 134
  stertorous 113
Brivaracetam 21, 33, 35, 36

C

Calcitonin gene-related peptide 135
Calcium 25
Cannabidiol 125, 134
Carbamazepine 6, 13, 17, 31, 35, 36, 42, 126
Cardiac bradyarrhythmia 83
Cardiomyopathy 45
Cardiovascular system 136
Cenobamate 26
Central nervous system 42
  infection 3
Centromedian nucleus 74, 85
Cerebellar stimulation 86, 87
Cerebellum 86
Cerebral folate deficiency 126
Cerebrospinal fluid 104, 128
Cerebrovascular disease 11
Chronic ambulatory electrocorticographic monitoring 89
Clobazam 14, 26, 32, 35, 125
Clonic movements 65
Cognitive behavioral
  outcomes 18
  therapy 116, 133
Cognitive dysfunction 40
Combination therapy 37
Combined oral contraceptive pills 19, 20
Computed tomography 3
Confusion, postictal 113
Constipation 45
Continuous
  electroencephalogram monitoring 100
  role of 100
Continuous positive airway pressure 83
  therapy 134

Index

Contraceptive 19, 20*fc*
  choices 21
  counseling 21
  pills, combined oral 19, 20
Copper histidine 126
CoQ10 deficiency syndromes 126
Cortical spreading depression 134
Cortical venous thrombosis 105
Cranial implantable pulse
    generator 79*f*
Creatine deficiency syndrome
  126
Cryptogenic focal epilepsy 49
Cytochrome p450 32

D

Deep brain stimulation 74, 79,
    83, 84
  management 85*fc*
  targets 83
Dementia 134
Depot medroxyprogesterone
    acetate 20
Depression 6, 24, 111, 134
Diabetes 45, 136
Diet
  arginine-restricted 126
  role of 44
  therapy 75
    type of 75
Diffusion tensor imaging 89
Diffusion-weighted imaging 67
Dizziness 13
Dravet syndrome 42, 124, 125
Drug-resistant epilepsy 35, 40,
    62, 71, 75, 79*f*
  medical management of 40
  surgical management in 71*fc*
  treatment of 73
Drugs 97, 98
  interactions 34, 36, 38
Dual-energy X-ray
    absorptiometry 25
Dysplastic brain tissue, resection
    of 72

E

Eclampsia 103
Electrical stimulation 79
  neuromodulatory effects of 79
  therapy 80
Electrocardiogram 3
Electroconvulsive therapy 84, 102

Electrocorticography 84
  chronic 89
  intraoperative 70
Electrode
  configuration 85
  implantation, target of 85
Electroencephalogram 4, 6, 30,
    50, 51, 56, 57, 59, 94, 127, 128,
    133
  abnormal 51, 52
Electroencephalographic
    monitoring 13
Electroencephalography 63, 66,
    71
  interictal 66, 68, 69
    high-resolution 68
  intracranial 70
Emergency surgery 102
Emotional dysregulation 111*f*
Encephalopathy 32
  developmental 126
  early infantile epileptic 123,
    126
  epileptic 49, 122, 126
Endocrine disorders 135
Enteric nervous system 135
Enzyme, hepatic 38
Epigastric rising sensation 65
Epilepsy 1, 9, 11, 12, 15, 18, 20,
    24, 30, 41, 44, 48, 49*b*, 51, 57,
    66, 73, 78, 80, 80*f*, 105, 117,
    122, 130, 132, 134, 136
  benign occipital 49
  catamenia 18
  childhood absence 49
  comorbidities 11, 130
  duration of 53
  early 4
  early-onset 14
  extratemporal lobe 56
  familial focal 123
  familial mesial temporal lobe
    123
  focal 51
  genetic 122-124, 125*f*
  generalized 49
  idiopathic generalized 13, 23
  juvenile
    absence 49, 57
    myoclonic 49, 57
  management 18, 36
  of infancy with migrating focal
    seizures 123, 126
  onset of 53
  pharmacoresistant 62
  pharmacotherapy of 45

  protocol magnetic resonance
    imaging 66
  pseudorefractory 63
  reading 49
  refractory 67, 81*t*
  self-limited infantile 123
  sleep-related hypermotor 123
  structural sequences,
    harmonized neuroimaging
    of 66, 71
  sudden unexpected death in 7,
    40, 78, 131
  surgery 55, 56*b*, 62, 66*t*, 68, 72
  surgical management of 68*t*
  syndrome 49*t*, 79*f*, 125, 126
  temporal lobe 56
  treatment of 137
  type of 34, 52
  uncontrolled 55
Epileptiform
  abnormalities 50, 53
  discharges, interictal 63
Epileptogenic lesion 63*f*
Episodes 104
Eslicarbazepine 33, 35, 36, 132
Essential tremor 84
Ethosuximide 33, 35, 125
Everolimus 126
Expressive language dysfunction
  36
Eye blinking 64

F

Fear 64
Febrile
  infection-related epilepsy
    syndrome 104
  seizures 53, 57, 123, 124
  seizures plus phenotype 124
Fenfluramine 26, 125
Fertility 24
Fibromyalgia 112, 135
Fluid-attenuated inversion
    recovery 67
Fluorodeoxyglucose 69
Focal cortical dysplasia 70, 72,
    123
Focal impaired awareness
    seizures 65
Folate metabolism 126
Folic acid 21
Folinic acid 126
Fosphenytoin 33, 94
Free thyroxine 21

Functional seizures 109, 110, 111*f*, 117
   evaluation of 116*t*
   management of 109, 112

G

Gabapentin 21, 35, 132
Gamma-aminobutyric acid 32, 43, 73, 87, 93, 95, 134
Ganaxolone 126
Gastrointestinal absorption 13
Gastrointestinal system 135
Gene 125, 126
Genetic epilepsy 122-124, 125*f*
   classification of 123, 123*f*, 124*t*
   management of 122, 124
Gestural automatisms 65
Gingival hypertrophy 36
Globus pallidus interna 84*f*
Glucose transporter 43
   deficiency 126
      syndrome 128
Glutamate 134
Glycine 126
Gonadotropin-releasing hormone 19
   analogs 19
Goserelin 19

H

Hair loss 36
Hamartoma, hypothalamic 73
Headache, postictal 66
Headiness 113
Heart disease 134
Hemimegalencephaly 73
Hemispherectomy, functional 73
Hemispherotomy 73
Hemorrhage 3
Hepatic enzyme inducers 38
High-resolution imaging 67
Hippocampal sclerosis 72
Hormone
   adrenocorticotropic 128
   replacement therapy 24, 24*t*
Hot flashes 24
Hybrid extraoperative electroencephalogram 70
Hyperglycemia 13
Hyperlipidemia 45
Hypertension 136
Hypnotherapy 116
Hypoglycemia 13, 45
Hyponatremia 36, 132
Hypothermia 103
Hypothesis formulation 64
Hypothyroidism 21
Hypoxic brain injury 3

I

Ictal electroencephalogram 66
Ictal single-photon-emission computed tomography 69
Ictal speech arrest 65
Immunoglobulin, intravenous 101
Immunomodulation, role of 101
Immunotherapy 101
Impaired cognitive function 23
Infantile epileptic spasms syndrome 122-124, 126
Inhalational halogenated anesthetics 99
Injuries 40
Integrated cognitive model 111*f*
Intellectual disability 23, 51
Intelligence quotient 59, 66
International League against Epilepsy 1, 64, 93, 122
Interpersonal therapy 116
Intrauterine device 20
Ion channels 125

K

Ketamine 96, 98
Ketogenic diet 43, 75, 102, 126
Kidney stones 36, 45

L

Lacosamide 14, 21, 26, 33, 35, 42, 132
Lamotrigine 6, 14, 17, 19, 32, 35, 36, 125, 132
Landau–Kleffner syndrome 126, 132
Laryngeal dysfunction 83
Laser interstitial thermal therapy 73
Lennox–Gastaut syndrome 42, 73, 126, 132
Levetiracetam 17, 31, 35, 36, 42, 94, 132
Lobectomy, temporal 57*b*
Low bone density 12
Low glycemic index treatment 75
Lysosomal storage disorders 123

M

Magnesium 103
   supplementation 105
Magnetic resonance imaging 3, 51, 56, 57, 59, 66, 71, 81, 83, 127, 128
   functional 68, 70, 71
   sequences 67*t*
Magnetoencephalography 63, 68, 69, 71
   interictal 68
Major congenital malformations 18, 23
Medical Research Council Antiepileptic Drug Withdrawal Group 50
Medium Chain Triglyceride diet 75
Medroxyprogesterone 19
Memantine 126
Menkes disease 126
Menopausal symptoms, management of 24
Menopause 24
Mesial temporal lobe epilepsy 72
Metabolic disorders, inherited 126
Midazolam 97
Migraine 36, 134
Mini-mental state examination 133
Misconception 66
Montreal cognitive assessment 133
Mood
   changes 24
   stabilization 36
Multiple seizure types 51
Multitarget deep brain stimulation 87

N

National Institute for Clinical Excellence 24
Neural tube defects 22
Neurocritical Care Society 96
Neurocysticercosis 58
Neurodevelopmental disorders 111, 126
Neurological deficit 51
Neurological disease, chronic 130
Neuromodulation 73
   mechanism of action in 79

techniques, summary of 74t
type of 73
Neuropsychiatric comorbidity 131
Neuropsychological tests 64, 115
Neurostimulation 78
   devices 79
   techniques 79f
   therapy 79f
Neurostimulator system 88f
Neutral antiseizure medications 21
Next-generation sequencing 127
Night sweats 24
N-methyl-D-aspartate 98, 126, 134
   receptors 95
Noninvasive transcranial direct cortical stimulation 86
Nonpharmacological treatment 44
Non-rapid eye movement sleep 134
Normothermia 103
Nose wiping, postictal 66

O

Obstructive sleep apnea 83, 133
Olfactory hallucinations 65
Opisthotonus 113b
Ornithine 126
Oxcarbazepine 17, 32, 35, 36, 42, 132

P

Pancreatitis, acute 45
Parempanel 14
Paresis, postictal 66
Parkinson's disease 84
Paroxysmal kinesigenic dyskinesia 126
Paroxysms, behavioral 111f
Patient data management system 88f
Pentobarbital 97
Peptic ulcer disease 134
Perampanel 26, 33, 35, 36
Periventricular nodular heterotopia 73
Personality disorders 111
Pharyngeal dysfunction 83
Phenobarbital 25, 134
Phenobarbitone 35

Phenytoin 6, 13, 25, 33, 35, 36, 42, 94, 132
Polycystic ovary syndrome 136
Polymicrogyria 73
Polytherapy 136
Positron emission tomography 68, 69, 71
   interictal 69
Posterior reversible encephalopathy syndrome 105
Postictal phenomenon 66, 66t
Post-traumatic stress disorder 25
Potassium channel 125
Preeclampsia 103
Pregabalin 21, 132
Pregnancy 21, 104
Progesterone 20, 24
Progestogen-only pill 20
Prolonged exposure technique 116
Propofol infusion syndrome 100
Pseudoseizures 110
Pseudosleep 113
Psychiatric dysfunction 40
Psychodynamic therapy 116
Psychological comorbidity
   evaluation of 115
   management of 115, 116
Psychological therapies 116
Psychological trauma 111
Psychopathology 111f
Psychopharmacologic agents 116
Psychotherapy, mindfulness-based 116
Pulse width 85
Pyridoxine 104, 126
   metabolism pathway 126
Pyruvate dehydrogenase deficiency 45

Q

Quinidine 125

R

Radiofrequency ablation 73
Randomized control trials 81, 133
Rapamycin, mammalian target of 43, 124
Rasmussen's encephalitis 49, 73
Rational antiseizure medications management, principles of 41

Rational polytherapy 41, 44
Refractoriness 94
Refractory status epilepticus 94, 95
   management of 93, 95, 101
   treatment of 97t
Repetitive transcranial magnetic stimulation 74, 101
Reproductive endocrine disorder 136
Responsive neurostimulation 72, 74, 79, 87
   clinical evidence for 88
Restless leg syndrome 133
Robotic thermocoagulative hemispherotomy 70
   concept of 70
Rolandic epilepsy, benign 49

S

Seizures 1, 6, 6fc, 9, 11, 30, 43, 44, 52, 64, 105, 110, 111f, 114
   absence 32
   acute symptomatic 2, 58
   behavior 112
   clinical manifestations of 12
   complex febrile 51
   control 21
   dacrystic 65
   daily 64
   dissociative 110
   early poststroke 11
   epileptic 109, 113b
   episode 1
   febrile 53, 57, 123, 124
   freedom, duration of 52, 53
   frequency 24
      estrogen-related 24
   functional 109, 110, 111f, 117
   gelastic 65
   higher risk of recurrence 51b, 56b
   history of 51
   hypermotor 65
   hysterical 110
   management 21, 30
   myoclonic 32, 51, 52
   nonconvulsive 13
   onset 52
   psychogenic 110
      nonepileptic 2, 13, 25, 63, 111f, 131
   recurrence 52
      risk of 50
      timing of 54

Index

scaffold 111f, 117
single 4
strong activation of 111f
tonic-clonic 3, 24, 32, 65, 136
type of 2, 34, 35, 35t, 52
unprovoked 2, 5
Selective serotonin reuptake inhibitors 25, 132
Self-limited epilepsy with centrotemporal spikes 5, 126
Sensing-enabled deep brain stimulation, new generation of 87
Sensory disturbances 65
Serine biosynthesis disorders 126
Serotonin and norepinephrine reuptake inhibitors 132
Sexual dysfunction 36
Single-photon-emission computed tomography 68, 69, 71
Sleep
  apnea 83
  disorders 133
S-licarbazepine 33
Slow wave sleep 134
Sodium channel 125
  blockers 126
Status epilepticus 3, 13, 40, 93, 104
  convulsive 95
  refractory 94, 95, 104
  severity score 94
  super refractory 101
Stereoelectroencephalography 68, 70, 71
Stevens–Johnson syndrome 32
Stimulation frequency 85
Stimulus, pulse width of 85
Stiripentol 125
Stroke, ischemic 3
Sturge–Weber syndrome 73

Subclavicular implantable pulse generator 79f
Substantia nigra 87
Subthalamic nucleus 84, 87
Sulfonylurea 126
Surgery 72, 73
Surgically remediable epilepsy syndromes 72
Susceptibility-weighted imaging 67

T

Thalamus
  anterior nucleus of 83, 85fc
  centromedian nucleus of 74
Thiopental 97
Thyroid
  disorders 21
  function, regular monitoring of 21
  hormones 136
  peroxidase antibodies levels 21
  stimulating hormone 21
Tongue bite 113
Tonic-clonic seizures
  bilateral 3
  generalized 24, 32, 65, 136
  presence of 52
Topiramate 6, 17, 33, 35, 36, 132
Toxic epidermal necrolysis 32
Transcranial direct current stimulation 74
Traumatic brain injury 3
Traumatic stress disorder 111
Traumatization 111f
Tricyclic antidepressants 25
Trigeminal nerve stimulation 74
Triptorelin 19
T-score 25
Tuberous sclerosis 126
  complex 72
Tumor necrosis factor alpha 135

U

Ubiquinone deficiency syndromes 126
Unilateral interictal epileptiform discharges 57
United States Food and Drug Administration 80
Unprovoked seizure 2, 5
  evaluation of 3
Urinary incontinence 113

V

Vagal nerve stimulation 73, 79-81, 83t, 133
Vaginal dryness 24
Vagus nerve stimulation 72, 74, 79, 81t, 83
  clinical evidence for 81
  responsive 83
Valproate 14, 17, 19, 32, 35, 36, 38, 125, 132
Valproic acid 32, 94
Versive movements 65
Video-electroencephalogram 66, 128
  monitoring 64, 114
    minimum duration of 64
Vigabatrin 35
Visual hallucinations 65
Vitamin D 25
Vomiting 45

W

Weight loss 36
World Health Organization 20

Z

Zeiler's systematic review 103
Zonisamide 21, 26, 34, 35